T5-AXO-730

Emergency Nutrition Assessment

Guidelines for field workers

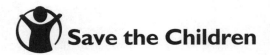
Save the Children

Save the Children UK is a member of the International Save the Children Alliance, the world's leading independent children's rights organisation, with members in 29 countries and operational programmes in more than 100.

Save the Children works with children and their communities to provide practical assistance and, by influencing policy and public opinion, bring about positive change for children.

Published by
Save the Children
1 St John's Lane
London EC1M 4AR
UK

First published 2004

© The Save the Children Fund 2004
Registered Charity No. 213890

ISBN 1 84187 090 0

All rights reserved. No reproduction, copy or transmission of this publication may be made without written permission, except under the terms set out below.

This publication is copyright, but may be reproduced by any method without fee or prior permission for teaching purposes, but not for resale. For copying in any other circumstances, prior written permission must be obtained from the publisher, and a fee may be payable.

Typeset by Avon DataSet Ltd, Bidford on Avon, Warwickshire B50 4JH

CONTENTS

Abbreviations

ACF	Action Contre la Faim
ARI	Acute respiratory infection
BMI	Body mass index
BCG	Anti-tuberculosis vaccination
CDC	Centers for Disease Control and Prevention
CI	Confidence interval
CMR	Crude mortality rate
CSAS	Centric systematic area sampling
DHS	Demographic and health surveys
EGS	Employment generation scheme
EPI	Expanded programme of immunisation
EWS	Early warning system
FAO	Food and Agriculture Organization
FEZ	Food economy zone
GFD	General food distribution
HEA	Household economy approach
HFA	Height-for-age
HH	Household
ICRC	International Committee of the Red Cross
IDA	Iron deficiency anaemia

IDD	Iodine deficiency disorders
IDP	Internally displaced person
MCH	Maternal and child health
MoA	Ministry of Agriculture
MoH	Ministry of Health
MSF	Médecins Sans Frontières
MUAC	Mid-upper arm circumference
NCHS	National Centre for Health Statistics
NGO	Non-governmental organisation
NSP	Nutrition surveillance programme
PDAR	Person days at risk
PWLH/A	People living with HIV/AIDS
SFP/SFC	Supplementary feeding programme/centre
SNNPR	Southern Nations, Nationalities and Peoples Region
TALC	Teaching Aids at Low Cost
TB	Tuberculosis
TFP/TFC	Therapeutic feeding programme/centre
UNHCR	United Nations High Commissioner for Refugees
U5MR	Under-five mortality rate
VAM	Vulnerability analysis and mapping
WFA	Weight-for-age

WFH   Weight-for-height

WFP   World Food Programme

WHM   Weight-for-height median

WHO   World Health Organization

WHZ   Weight-for-height z-score

Introduction

This manual is intended to provide straightforward and comprehensive guidance to nutritionists and other field workers who are responsible for conducting assessments in emergency settings. It is hoped that it will contribute to improving practice by providing step-by-step guidance, taking the practitioner from the theory through to the practice of conducting an assessment and producing a report.

The term *assessment* rather than *survey* is used deliberately. An anthropometric survey and mortality survey form part of an emergency nutrition assessment. However, an assessment also includes the gathering of information to understand the causes of malnutrition. In the absence of a sound understanding of causes, it is impossible to interpret the prevalence of malnutrition and the rate of mortality found in the surveys. It is also impossible to develop appropriate recommendations.

The prevalence of malnutrition and rate of mortality are increasingly used by international agencies to compare the extent of human suffering in different parts of the world in order to prioritise the use of resources. It is therefore of utmost importance that this data is collected using sound methods, presented in a transparent manner and interpreted meaningfully in light of information about the causes of malnutrition.

Currently, nutrition assessments are often little more than anthropometric surveys where the focus is on delivering the malnutrition prevalence figure. Furthermore, in many instances, standard methodologies for gathering representative data are not followed. This means that even the validity of the prevalence figure is thrown into doubt. Finally, nutrition interventions in emergencies are typically narrow in focus and tend to concentrate on treating malnutrition. Anthropometric surveys are therefore often conducted to validate programme decisions to open or close feeding programmes rather than inform a broader set of possible decisions to address the causes of malnutrition.

This manual is intended to help overcome some of these problems. A major part of the manual is devoted to assessing the causes of malnutrition and interpreting this information alongside mortality and malnutrition information. In addition, the steps involved in conducting an anthropometric survey are laid out for the beginner with clear guidance on the rules, which should be followed and those which can be adapted for different contexts. The manual draws on Save the Children's experience, highlighted in numerous examples in the text, and our understanding of common mistakes, challenges in analysis and interpretation. This guidance is supported by a new set of tools to assist with survey design and analysis, which are on the CD-ROM that accompanies the manual. The recommendations in this manual are consistent with the Sphere Minimum Standards for Disaster Response and make close reference to the standard on food security and nutrition assessment and analysis (The Sphere Project, 2004).

We envisage that this manual could be used in a number of specific circumstances. First, and most obvious, is to assess the nutritional situation in an emergency-affected population with a view to identifying responses which address the real need and contribute to the realisation of the human rights of the population. Second, nutrition assessments are frequently conducted with the aim of monitoring the situation in order to inform the ongoing design of interventions and determine whether a programme is effective or not. This manual provides some guidance on the latter activity, although it concentrates on the former.

As the title indicates, the manual is intended for use in emergency situations when a shock has occurred that is affecting the health situation, people's access to food or their capacity to care for one another. In the chapters devoted to estimating the prevalence of malnutrition we focus on the measurement of acute rather than chronic malnutrition. This means that the manual will have limited value in development settings though it may provide a useful framework for assessing long-term causes of malnutrition and conducting a representative survey. However, development settings often require more complex survey designs if, for example, baseline data is being gathered or project impact is being assessed.

The book is divided into six major parts. Part A provides guidelines on how to conduct an assessment of the causes of malnutrition in an emergency. This involves gathering and analysing secondary data, identifying the primary data that is required and the most appropriate methods for gathering it, and finally, analysing the data and developing a locally specific analysis of causes.

Part B provides guidelines on the anthropometric survey, taking the reader from basic information on anthropometric indicators to analysis and presentation of the findings. This part should be used alongside Save the Children's guidelines on the use of Epi Info for Data processing and Analysis of Anthropometric Aurveys (Save the Children, 2003). Those guidelines are on the CD-ROM attached to this manual.[1]

Part C provides guidelines on how to conduct a retrospective mortality survey, recognising that this is often done alongside an anthropometric survey. It describes some of the principles of measuring mortality and alternative methodologies for gathering the data. It also provides guidance on analysing and presenting the data.

Part D focuses on how to interpret the data which results from working through parts A–C. It provides guidance on how to judge the seriousness of a situation and how to develop recommendations. It also provides an outline for a model nutrition assessment report.

---

[1] New software is being developed for analysis of nutrition surveys and is available for testing on www.nutrisurvey.de

Part E contains a practical checklist of tasks which need to be carried out from the beginning to the end of the assessment. It also provides information about training the team and ensuring the quality of data collected in the field.

Part F addresses the situation where nutrition assessments are used to monitor or evaluate a humanitarian response or where nutrition assessments are used to measure the coverage of a feeding programme.

Appendix 9 provides a glossary of key terms.

This manual comes with a CD-ROM that includes electronic versions of a number of the key texts referred to in the manual. In addition, it provides a set of tools which can assist with the design and analysis of the assessment findings. For example, there are simple tools for calculating required sample sizes and spreadsheets for easily calculating confidence intervals for mortality rates.

Save the Children UK welcomes comments on this manual so that any future editions can be improved.

Acknowledgements

This manual has benefited from major contributions from our three reviewers: Bradley A. Woodruff, Mark Myatt and Helen Young, who have provided enormous guidance from broad conceptual issues down to minute detail. We sincerely thank them for giving their experience, expertise and support so generously. Save the Children, however, takes full responsibility for the manual's contents. Mark Myatt is behind the development of almost all the tools on the CD-ROM and has also been the key developer of some of the new methodologies presented in this manual. We would also like to thank Andrew Tomkins for his particular contribution to the section on infection and malnutrition and Sarah Richards for the review she conducted in preparation for drafting.

This manual originates from one developed by the Nutrition Guideline Working Group for the Disaster Prevention and Preparedness Commission in Ethiopia. While the manual looks quite different now, we gratefully acknowledge the sound draft that we began with, which was the result of months of work by the Working Group.

We also acknowledge that this manual draws heavily on other manuals, although we do, of course, hope it brings some additional guidance and makes a significant contribution to the literature. We specifically would like to note our substantive reference to the MSF Nutrition Guidelines, draft 2000, the Action Contre la Faim's *Assessment and Treatment of Malnutrition in Emergency Situations*, the WFP *Food and Nutrition Handbook*, the WHO *The Management of Nutrition in Major Emergencies* and Helen Young and Susan Jaspar's *Nutrition Matters*. To avoid repeated referencing throughout the text we have not acknowledged our reference to these texts throughout.

Arabella Duffield and Anna Taylor were responsible for writing the manual.

Part A
Assessing the causes of malnutrition

This part of the manual is intended to guide you through the steps required to conduct a context-specific analysis of the causes of malnutrition. Use this analysis to help you interpret the information you collect during the anthropometric and mortality surveys. Any interpretation of nutrition assessment findings must involve examining the prevalence of malnutrition, the mortality rate and the causes of malnutrition together in order to draw conclusions about the situation and make recommendations for any intervention required (this is described in Chapter D1).

The first chapter begins with a brief discussion of the different types of malnutrition. This is followed by a theoretical overview of the Unicef conceptual framework of the causes of malnutrition, because it provides the foundation for developing a context-specific analysis. Subsequent chapters take you through the various steps required to undertake a causal analysis (see page 18). These are organised in the order in which they should be undertaken, starting with the review of secondary data and ending with the development of a context-specific causal analysis with the major causes identified.

Chapter A1
Introduction to the causes of malnutrition

A1.1 The Unicef conceptual framework of the causes of malnutrition

The Unicef conceptual framework (Figure A1.1) has become widely used as a tool to examine the causes of malnutrition since the early 1990s. The framework clearly shows that malnutrition has many causes and is not solely related to food. It is essential to understand the different reasons why malnutrition has developed in the emergency-affected population before designing any interventions to address malnutrition.

The Unicef framework is organised into three layers of causes which contribute to the ultimate outcome of a malnourished individual (at the top of the framework). These layers of causal factors operate at different levels of society. Immediate causes operate at the individual level, underlying causes operate at household or community level, and basic causes operate at the community, national and global level.

A1.2 What is malnutrition?

Before considering the causes on the framework, it is necessary to consider the outcome of interest at the top of the framework: malnutrition. Adequate nutrition is the means by which people thrive, maintain growth, resist and recover from diseases and perform their daily tasks. When nutrition is inadequate, people become malnourished. Common consequences of malnutrition[1] include growth failure, deficiency in specific micronutrients, decreased resistance to disease and reduced ability to work. Pregnancy and lactation may also be affected.

The two manifestations of malnutrition which we are particularly concerned about in emergency situations is weight loss (often combined with growth failure in children or failure to gain weight in pregnancy) and micronutrient deficiency. Marasmus and kwashiorkor result from deficiencies in multiple nutrients and, while present in many poor countries, can become more widespread during emergencies. Marasmus is characterised by wasting

---

[1] Malnutrition includes over-nutrition (obesity) and under-nutrition. These guidelines focus exclusively on under-nutrition as this is by far the most common type of malnutrition in emergencies. Therefore malnutrition means under-nutrition in these guidelines.

Figure A1.1 The Unicef conceptual model of the causes of malnutrition

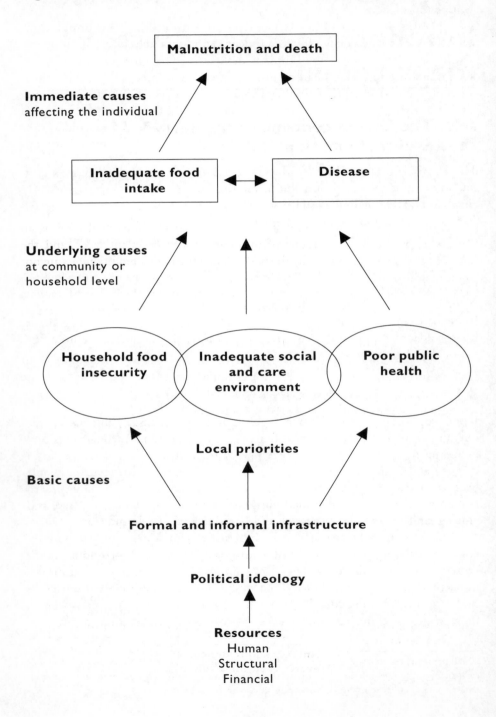

and kwashiorkor by nutritional oedema, although these conditions have many other clinical signs.

Specific micronutrient deficiencies are widespread in populations which are not emergency affected. Indeed, approximately two billion people worldwide suffer from some kind of deficiency. The most common deficiencies are due to a lack of iron (iron deficiency anaemia – IDA), vitamin A (xerophthalmia) and iodine (iodine deficiency disorders [IDD] including goitre and cretinism). However, outbreaks of other types of deficiency have occurred in emergencies among populations entirely dependent on food aid. These include deficiencies of vitamin C (scurvy), niacin (pellagra), thiamine (beriberi) and riboflavin.

A1.3 Immediate causes

The immediate cause of malnutrition, operating at the individual level, is an imbalance between the amount of nutrients absorbed by the body and the amount of nutrients required by the body. When the body's requirements are not met, malnutrition can occur. This happens as a consequence of consuming too little food or having an infection which either increases the body's requirements or causes the body not to absorb the food consumed. In practice, these two problems often occur at the same time because one can lead to another. This is illustrated in the infection and malnutrition cycle shown in Figure A1.2.

Most mortality in the initial period of an emergency is caused by four infectious diseases: gastro-enteritis (for example, shigellosis and cholera), acute lower respiratory infections, measles and malaria. These diseases often occur alongside malnutrition (Moren, 1995; Toole and Waldman, 1990).

Different infections interact differently with nutrition. The interaction depends on the infection itself and on the extent of malnutrition. Table A1.1 shows how the major diseases in emergencies interact with nutrition. In general terms, poor nutrition can result in reduced immunity to infection – this can

Figure A1.2 The malnutrition/infection cycle (adapted from Tomkins and Watson, 1989)

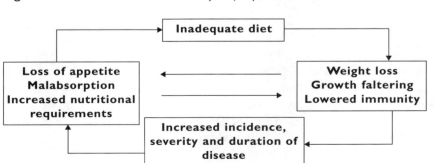

increase the likelihood of an individual getting the infection, or increase its duration or severity. Infection in turn can result in loss of appetite or an increase in nutritional requirements or a loss of nutrients from the body in the case of diarrhoea. This triggers further weight loss, resulting once again in reduced resistance to further infection.

Table A1.1 Summary table of interactions between malnutrition and the major killers in emergencies

	Impact of malnutrition on infection	Impact of infection on factors leading to malnutrition
Diarrhoea (eg, shigellosis)	• Increased duration • Increased severity • Increased mortality	• Malabsorption • Appetite loss • Losses of endogenous nutrients
ARI (lower)	• Increased severity • Increased mortality	• Appetite loss • Metabolic effects resulting in muscle breakdown
Measles	• Increased duration • Increased severity • Increased mortality	• Appetite loss • Decreased levels of plasma vitamin A • Prolonged immune suppression resulting in increased incidence of ARI and diarrhoea • Fever increasing requirements* • Metabolic effects resulting in muscle breakdown
Malaria	• Some evidence of increased severity in deficiencies of vitamin A and zinc	• Anaemia • Impaired foetal development, low birth weight and growth faltering

*Severely malnourished individuals may not experience a fever.

As with other infections, HIV/AIDS interacts with malnutrition to form a vicious cycle. When an individual has HIV but is asymptomatic their energy requirements increase by 10%. This increases to 30% when they become symptomatic (WHO, 2003). If someone has HIV/AIDS, having a good nutritional status (without micronutrient deficiency) protects them against opportunistic infections; a reduction in opportunistic infections in turn protects them against nutritional deterioration. Opportunistic infections which can result in weight loss are oral thrush and mouth sores, which can make eating very painful, and persistent diarrhoea, which can lead to substantial nutrient losses. Diet is also an important determinant of the success or failure of HIV/AIDS drug regimens due to food and drug interactions.

A1.4 Underlying causes

Whether an individual gets enough food to eat or whether s/he is at risk of infection is mainly the result of factors operating at household and community level. These are known in the framework as the underlying causes. They are grouped into three types: those related to food security, those related to the social and care environment, and those related to public health.

Food security

Food security exists when all people, at all times, have physical and economic access to sufficient, safe and nutritious food for a healthy and active life (The Sphere Project, 2004, p. 108). Therefore, people are only food secure when food is both available and accessible; in other words, not only must it be available on the market, but it must also be affordable to people. For an active and healthy life, people need not only enough kilocalories to eat but also protein, fat and micronutrients. Food security encompasses both the quantity and the quality of food accessed. People are only food secure if they can meet their food needs all through the year. Marginalisation (political, economic, ethnic) of groups as well as the intra-household dynamics of food distribution determine whether all people are food secure.

People pursue a variety of livelihood strategies in order to achieve food security. A livelihood strategy is the combination of activities which households undertake, usually in a specific geographical area, to make ends meet. Broad livelihood strategies may include agro-pastoralism, fishing and hunting, pastoralism, and a variety of employment-based strategies.[2] Within the same livelihood zone,[3] different households have different degrees of wealth, which means that some are more food secure than others.

Food security is increasingly being considered within a broader 'sustainable livelihoods' framework, which assists in understanding the range of economic, social, institutional and political factors and processes that ultimately determine livelihood outcomes.

The framework highlights the range of factors that determine livelihood outcomes, and the dynamic relationships between them (rather than any simple causal relationship). The strategies that households pursue, and the extent to which they are successful in ensuring food security, depend on three broad sets of factors:

---

[2] These broad strategies may be sub-divided further. For example, Somalia has several different pastoral livelihood groups, some keeping camels and goats, and selling animals to markets in the Gulf, some keeping cattle and sheep, and selling their animals to Kenya.

[3] A livelihood or food economy zone is a geographical area over which people pursue similar livelihood strategies such as agro-pastoralism. Food economy or livelihood zones are usually geographically distinct but they may not be; for example, there may be a rice farming zone covered with small zones where fishing is the main livelihood strategy.

Figure A1.3 Sustainable livelihoods framework

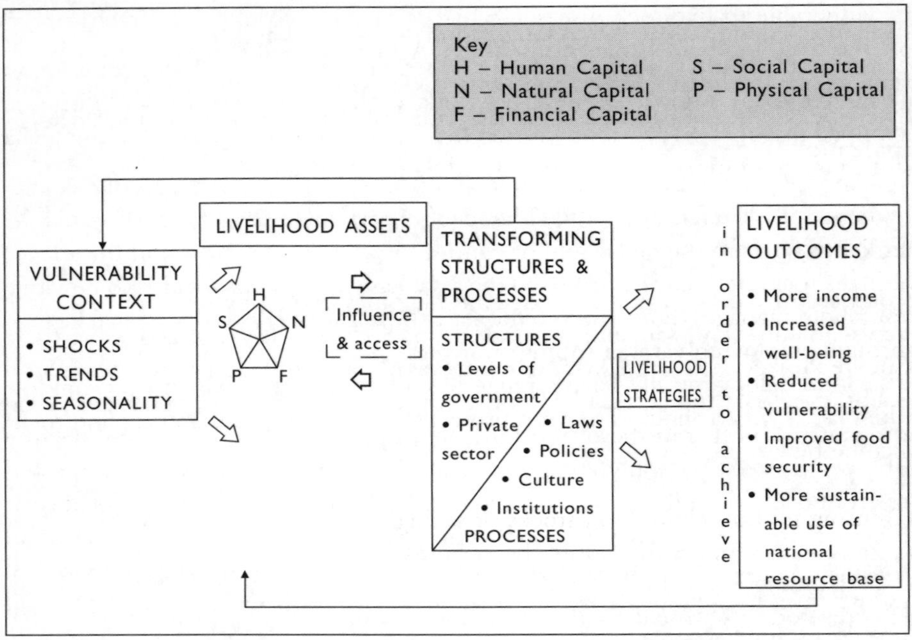

Source: DFID Sustainable Livelihoods Guidance Sheets; www.livelihoods.org

- their asset base: including tangible types of capital/assets such as land, livestock and cash saving, and less tangible types such as the skills and education of household members, and their links to social and kinship networks
- structures and processes: the legal, political and cultural factors that influence both access to assets and the ways in which those assets can be put to use
- the vulnerability context: the external environment in which people exist.

The framework could be viewed as an elaboration of the 'household food insecurity' group of causes on the Unicef conceptual framework. The actual livelihood strategies pursued (and to some extent the asset base within the household) determine the quantity and quality of food available for household members and thus can contribute to the underlying causes of malnutrition. The external asset base, the structure and processes, and the vulnerability context usually constitute the basic causes of malnutrition which determine the sorts of livelihood strategies which can be pursued. These basic causes can also contribute to the social and care environment and public health (see below).

An understanding of livelihood strategies and patterns of access to food and income helps us to understand households' and communities' vulnerability in an emergency. Vulnerability includes both exposure and sensitivity to livelihood shocks (Devereux, 2002). For example, a pastoral community will be vulnerable to livestock diseases, which may have little or no direct impact on the livelihoods of urban households. A rich pastoralist household may be very reliant on livestock for food, whereas a poor pastoralist may have more diversified sources of food and be less vulnerable to a severe livestock disease epidemic.

Another way of considering vulnerability is through the concepts of risk and resilience. Risk refers to the likelihood of a particular shock occurring, while resilience refers to the household or community's ability to withstand the effects of that shock. Resilience is linked to the asset base of the household, and how the household manages those assets to mitigate the negative effects of external factors through employing various coping strategies.

Households typically have a range of coping strategies which they employ when faced with a shock. They can protect their consumption and expand their income by:

- using up household food stocks or savings
- receiving support from other households
- expanding some forms of normal income generation such as the sale of firewood or charcoal, or the collection of wild foods
- selling assets – the value of these assets will depend on their price relative to that of food.

In addition, households can cut back on their consumption by:

- reducing their food intake
- consuming cheaper, less desirable foods
- reducing expenditure on non-food items such as soap, clothing and healthcare
- reducing the number of dependent people in the household, eg, by sending young children away to relatives.

These coping strategies may impact on malnutrition differently. For example, reducing food intake may have a direct effect and sending a child to a relative may result in breastfeeding being curtailed. Expanding the sale of firewood may result in less time being spent on childcare, which could have a knock-on effect on child food intake.

Many of these strategies are part of normal seasonal variations, reflecting the different local needs and opportunities at different times of the year. Knowing when these normal and sustainable strategies are becoming stretched and even damaging to household current and future well-being is a critical aspect of understanding food security and nutrition. In an emergency, when the food security situation deteriorates drastically, the priorities of the individual and community shift towards survival. At this stage, coping mechanisms become more extreme and damaging for the household or individual. Inevitably, actions taken to avoid complete destitution become more and more irreversible: desperate actions such as the wholesale slaughter of productive animals have very serious consequences for future production.

The social and care environment

The social and care environment is the group of factors which affect the extent to which household members receive the care they need. The care environment determines whether the food available to household members and their potential for good health is translated into adequate food intake and prevention of disease. The care environment includes feeding practices (specifically breastfeeding and complementary feeding), hygiene and health-seeking practices, cognitive stimulation and psycho-social care for children and the care of women, especially adolescent girls, pregnant and lactating women. All of these caring practices require both time and other resources, demonstrating the link between these causes and the food security and public health causes, and the basic causes at the bottom of the framework.

The social environment refers to the broader social context of the household within the community and beyond (human and social capital assets in the sustainable livelihoods framework). It therefore encompasses social networks of support and the status of the household, including kinship networks. It also includes the role and educational status of women in communities and the extent to which they control resources in the household.

HIV/AIDS is widely acknowledged to have a major impact on the social and care environment. It can impact on direct caring behaviours, as traditional caregivers become chronically ill and require care themselves. This means that children or elderly people may become the principal care givers. It can also impact on the social environment. Stigma can affect people's relationships with other community members and the extent to which people can access social support mechanisms and basic services.

Public health

Public health is the group of factors relating to the health environment and therefore exposure to disease and access to basic health services. The health environment is affected by access to potable water and sanitation, the presence of malaria breeding sites, the quality of shelter and consequent level of cold, stress, overcrowding and the health of fellow community members, eg, whether they have been immunised or received anti-helminths recently.

Access to basic health services determines the extent to which infection can be prevented or treated. Effective treatment should reduce the duration and severity of infection. This can be particularly important for preventing the negative effects of infection on nutrition status (see Section A1.3). Access to health services is determined by their distance and cost (both direct, in terms of paying for treatment or transport, and indirect, in terms of the opportunity cost of attending). Poor-quality health services can create disincentives for uptake.

Links between underlying causes

In practice, the three groups of underlying causes overlap considerably. For example, imagine a child who has an infection. The time available to a mother to take her child to the nearest clinic depends on whether she is able to spare a day from working in the fields. While typically *time available for caring* would be considered a cause related to the social and care environment, in this instance the availability of time is affected by the extent of the household's food security, and how close the nearest clinic is. Thus, there are in fact at least three underlying reasons why this child is malnourished:

- (in the food security group of causes) is the lack of labour at household level resulting in severe time constraints on the carer
- (in the social and care environment group of causes) is the lack of time available for ensuring the health of the child
- (in the public health group of causes) is the distance to the nearest health facilities.

As a consequence of all of these factors, the child may experience a prolonged period of infection which results in appetite loss and failure to put on adequate weight (the immediate cause of malnutrition).

A1.5 Basic causes

As illustrated in Figure A1.1, the basic causes of malnutrition are a result of the resources available (human, structural and financial) and the political ideology affecting how these resources are used, particularly how they determine the formal and informal infrastructure which is put into place. Local priorities in turn determine to what extent households and communities can access these resources. The basic causes articulated in the sustainable livelihoods framework are the structures and processes, the vulnerability context and to some extent the assets (especially natural and physical assets) which determine livelihood outcomes.

The basic causes of malnutrition can be thought of as the real reasons behind the underlying causes. Consider the following underlying causes and possible basic causes.

Example underlying cause: Pastoralists have to sell livestock and cut back on milk intake due to drought which resulted in a deterioration in pasture.
Possible basic causes:

- inadequate veterinary services resulting in small livestock herds
- deterioration of the environment resulting in repeated drought years
- conflict has limited the areas which they can exploit for pasture.

Example underlying cause: Health services are not functioning.
Possible basic causes:

- the Ministry of Health has a tiny budget
- the numbers of health staff are reduced due to the consequences of HIV/AIDS
- all the available funds for health are spent on vertical programmes delivering specific inputs.

Example underlying cause: Women typically fail to exclusively breastfeed.
Possible basic causes:

- the status of women in society means they have a heavy workload immediately after pregnancy
- women receive little support from health services to breastfeed
- multinational companies are promoting the use of alternatives to breast-milk
- cultural barriers to exclusive breast feeding.

Each of these possible basic causes can be related to the resources available, the political ideology prevailing, the formal and informal infrastructure in place, and local priorities. In an emergency the most important basic cause to consider is the shock which has caused the emergency to occur. While it may not be possible to change the basic causes within the context of an emergency, their identification is important as it may highlight areas for advocacy or long-term intervention. Basic causes may also determine the nature of intervention at the underlying causes level. For example, a restocking intervention for pastoralists may cause more long-term nutritional vulnerability to drought if measures are not taken simultaneously to address environmental degradation.

The nature of the shock or shocks is critically important. It is not possible to give an exhaustive typology of possible shocks and their impacts. As referred to in Section A1.4, the extent to which a household or community is affected by a shock will depend on their vulnerability to it. A shock that can have particularly dramatic impact on nutrition is displacement resulting from the exhaustion of coping mechanisms or from conflict. In the absence of humanitarian relief, displacement often results in:

- people having little or no access to food
- the care environment being disrupted as people are separated from one another and livelihood strategies are totally upset
- a major change in public health, as people are often trying to survive with inadequate access to water in crowded unsanitary environments and in the absence of basic preventive health services.

A1.6 The seasonal dimension

Throughout the year the underlying, and therefore the immediate, causes of malnutrition change. All three groups of underlying causes are subject to seasonal variation. For example, access to food typically reduces prior to the harvest when workload is also high (for agricultural producers), or prior to the rains when workload finding water and pasture is high (for pastoralists). The health environment changes according to the temperature and rainfall. The care environment changes as labour requirements alter according to the agricultural cycle. This dynamic cannot be easily captured on the causal framework but special attention needs to be paid to this throughout the steps outlined in the next chapter.

Summary

- In order for nutrition interventions to be effective, the causes of malnutrition must be understood.
- The Unicef conceptual framework should be used to assess the causes of malnutrition when undertaking an emergency nutrition assessment. This means assessing:
  - the immediate causes of malnutrition, which are inadequate food intake and disease
  - the underlying causes of malnutrition, which are inadequate household food security and a poor public health, social and care environment
  - the basic causes of malnutrition, including a description of the shock itself.

CHAPTER A2

- Collect and review secondary information that already exists on malnutrition and its causes
- Check your secondary information for accuracy and relevance
- Systematically record secondary information

CHAPTER A3

- Construct a causal framework of malnutrition with the non-biased secondary information for before and after the emergency
- Construct a seasonal calendar with a timeline into the months following the assessment
- Identify gaps in your analysis

CHAPTER A4

- Develop a primary data collection plan based on the gaps in your analysis
- Decide which methods to use for data collection according to the type of data needed (further secondary data collection in the field, quantitative or qualitative collection of primary data)
- Prepare your data collection tools (questionnaires, checklists, discussion topics etc) to obtain this information

CHAPTER A5

- Analyse data where possible in the field
- Use your newly collected information to re-construct the causal analysis of malnutrition (pre and post emergency) and seasonal calendar
- Determine which causes result from the emergency and pose the greatest nutritional risk
- Identify gaps in your analysis

Chapter A2
Collecting and reviewing secondary information

The first step in developing the causal framework involves reviewing the secondary literature about the affected population. You will need to review secondary data which refers to the situation before and after the emergency. This secondary literature is then used to compile a pre-assessment causal framework (see Chapter A3).

This chapter is divided into four sections taking you through the main issues to consider in the review of secondary data:

1) what sort of information you are looking for
2) where information can be found
3) methods for reviewing the data
4) recording information during the review.

A2.1 Information you should look for

A2.1.1 Rates of malnutrition and mortality before the emergency

Gathering information on the prevalence of malnutrition and rate of mortality before the emergency is very useful for the following reasons.

- It can help you to interpret the likely impact of new causes of malnutrition. For example, when the typhoon hit Orissa in India in 1999 the rates of acute malnutrition in Orissa state from surveys conducted a couple of years previously were approaching 20%. There was no reason to suppose that these rates did not apply to the population when the typhoon struck. It was clear from this knowledge that even if there were only a small deterioration in the underlying causes of malnutrition, rates of malnutrition were already extremely high and were likely to be associated with excess mortality.
- It can help you to interpret the prevalence of malnutrition which results from your anthropometric survey (see Chapter D1 for more on this point).

You also need information on micronutrient deficiencies. In general, you can assume that if a population suffers from a micronutrient deficiency before an emergency, it is likely that the problem will remain afterwards. Therefore, secondary sources should be checked to find out the extent of these deficiencies before the emergency (see subsection A2.1.3 below as well).

A2.1.2 Immediate causes

Health status

In your review of secondary information on the public health situation, your most immediate concern should be recent or current outbreaks of disease that may be contributing to excess mortality and/or malnutrition. Outbreaks can worsen the nutritional situation but can of course also cause excess mortality. As indicated in Section A1.3 the main diseases of concern are diarrhoea, acute respiratory infection (ARI), measles and malaria. Epidemics of measles and shigella (SD1) will have a direct impact on the nutrition status of the population. Malaria may also affect nutritional status but is likely to have a major impact on mortality if a population is displaced from a non-endemic area to an area where malaria is endemic. ARI can be widespread in hot or cold and dusty environments. Information on which diseases are most common will help you interpret your rates of malnutrition and mortality (see Chapters A5 and D1).

You should seek to answer the following questions in your review of secondary information:

- Are there any reports of disease outbreaks which may affect nutritional status, eg, measles, acute diarrhoeal disease or malaria?
- Is the outbreak increasing or decreasing?
- Are there reports of high rates of ARI?
- Is there a high prevalence of HIV/AIDS or tuberculosis (TB) already making people vulnerable to malnutrition?
- Are there any endemic diseases, ie, diseases which happen every year at a particular time of year?

Food intake

You should review any information available on food intake. Food intake data is notoriously difficult to gather accurately (Gibson, 1990). However, it may be possible to find information which sheds light on intra-household food allocation and how decisions are made on who eats first at home. Some surveys might have gathered information on young child feeding practices and recorded the food reported to have been given to the child in the last 24 hours.

In this review you should seek to answer the following questions:

- How do people decide how to allocate food within the household? Who is likely to get the least food or the food of the poorest quality?

---

[1] Remember to examine the definition of a meal.

- What are young children typically fed and how frequent are their meals?
- How many meals[1] are different groups of the population reported to be eating? (This information would not be sufficient to determine food intake, but may shed light on the food security situation if there is data from another time to compare it with.)

A2.1.3 Food security information

Food security

Food security and livelihood assessments should provide you with the information about whether or not a shock, or the emergency, has caused deterioration in the population's food security situation. The analytical process is described in Figure A2.1.

Save the Children UK normally uses the household economy approach to get food security information and determine appropriate responses to address food insecurity. Household economy is defined as the sum of the ways in which a household gets its income, its savings and asset holdings, and its consumption of food and non-food items. The approach is described in detail in the Save the Children UK publication *The Household Economy Approach: A resource manual for practitioners.*[2]

A Household Economy Approach (HEA) explores how typical households from different wealth groups in a given area live in a normal (non-shock) year – this is known as an HEA baseline. Having this baseline description and understanding, it is then possible to judge how households may be able to cope with a shock or shocks using their own strategies and resources. Where appropriate, this involves predicting food aid needs and/or recommending other interventions to address household food insecurity.

You may need to use another agency's food security assessment if no HEA is available.

Other agencies may use different techniques to obtain food security information: for example, Oxfam uses the livelihood approach to assess food security and the International Federation for the Red Cross and Red Crescent Societies (IFRC) assesses economic security.

Most food security methodologies currently focus on the ways in which people access food and income and their overall levels of food security and/or poverty. In doing so, they typically go into more detail on tangible factors influencing food security, particularly financial, physical and natural capital, while also describing the vulnerability context. However, there is usually much less attention given to social capital, structures and processes. With the

---

[2] Available on the CD-ROM with this manual or to order from www.savethechildren.org/foodsecurity/publications

Figure A2.1   Food security assessment: the analytical process

---

1. The baseline or reference picture: How do people normally live?

   – How do households in common livelihood and wealth groups 'typically obtain their food and case income, and what is the relative importance of these different sources;
   – What are their connections with the market and with social or kinship networks;
   – What are their asset levels (food stocks normally carried over; livestock holdings; cash savings/capital; etc.); and
   – Normal expenditure patterns.

2. Defining the shock/s? What event/s have disrupted people's lives?

The sum of information about changes in the larger economy that will affect production and exchange options e.g. crop production 70–80% of normal; grain prices 120–130% of normal; people displaced from land

3. What is the initial impact of the shock and how are/will people cope?

   i) *Calculating the initial deficit/impact* – how does the shock affect different livelihood and wealth groups, according to their normal access to food and income, and the timing of the shock and subsequent activities?

   ii) *Calculating people's response to make up the initial impact* – how can or are the different livelihood and wealth groups respond/ing to the impact of the shock/s, according to their available coping strategies?

4. Results or outcome: what is the situation after the shock?

   • Are the different livelihood and wealth groups able to meet their basic food energy needs? If not, what is the estimated scale of the shortfall for these different groups?
   • Have dietary patterns changed, in terms of quality and variety, from normal, seasonal variations? If so how?
   • What types of coping strategies are being employed and are they considered relatively normal or sustainable, or likely to be harmful or damaging?
   • What are the timing implications of the shock/s and the nutrition survey? What are the anticipated changes in food security conditions in the coming months according to the seasonal opportunities and threats?

increased focus on the impact of HIV/AIDS, increasing importance is being given to looking at human capital and, to a lesser extent, social capital.

Whatever type of food security assessment you are reviewing, however, you need to be able to answer the following questions in order to assess the impact of food security on nutrition in the affected population:

- Is any part of the population facing a food deficit? If so, who? When will the deficit be experienced?
- What is the overall quality of the diet of different population groups? Is there access to foods of high dietary quality such as meat, milk, eggs, beans, oil, sugar and green leafy vegetables? If the population is dependent on relief food, is the ration adequate?
- Are people adopting or likely to adopt coping strategies which will have a negative effect on nutritional status (see Section A1.4)?
- Which periods of the year are likely to pose the greatest risk of childhood malnutrition? (For example, which periods of the year are busiest for the carers, when is food access most difficult, when will household demography change and have a knock-on effect on the social and care environment?)

Risk of micronutrient deficiency

If a population has access to a range of foods including staples (cereals or tubers), pulses or animal products, vitamin- and mineral-rich foods and fat sources, then the micronutrient requirements of the population should be met, provided adequate public health measures are in place to prevent diseases such as measles, malaria and parasitic infection. However, new micronutrient deficiencies do arise (other than those which are endemic) in populations which are dependent on food aid. Typically these include pellagra, beriberi, scurvy and riboflavin deficiency (see Section A1.2).

You should seek to answer the following questions in your review of secondary data to find out if the population is at risk of these deficiencies:

- Is there access to vitamin C-rich or fortified foods or appropriate supplements?
- Is there access to additional sources of niacin (eg, pulses, nuts, dried fish) if the staple is maize or sorghum?
- Is there access to additional sources of thiamine (eg, pulses, nuts, eggs) if the staple is polished rice?
- Is there access to adequate sources of riboflavin where people are dependent on a very limited diet?
- Are there cases of scurvy, pellagra, beriberi or riboflavin deficiency reported (see Table A2.1 below)?

Table A2.1 Key symptoms for selected micronutrient deficiencies

Beriberi (Thiamine)	• Wet beriberi: anorexia, ill-defined malaise associated with heaviness of legs, increase in pulse rate, complaints of pins and needles. Later signs include oedema spreading from legs to trunk, restlessness and rapid pulse rate and palpitations • Dry beriberi: early signs are similar to wet beriberi. Later signs include polyneuropathy (general dysfunction of nervous system) and muscles become progressively more wasted and walking becomes difficult
Scurvy (Vitamin C)	• Swollen and bleeding gums, minute haemorrhages around hair follicles leading to sheet haemorrhages on limbs, brittle hair, slow healing of wounds, infants tend to scream and lie on their backs in 'frog position' due to pain of limbs, progressive fatigue and pain in the limbs
Pellagra (Niacin)	• Deficiency affects the skin, gastro-intestinal tract and nervous system, therefore known as '3Ds': dermatitis, diarrhoea and dementia • Skin irritation occurring on sun-exposed areas of neck known as 'Cassal's necklace', redness and itching of skin or 'crazy paving' • Complaints of digestive system include nausea and constipation • Disturbances of the nervous system may cause depression, delirium (acute) or dementia (chronic)
Riboflavin deficiency (Vitamin B2)	• Angular stomatitis • Magenta tongue • 'Gritty' eyes

Relief food

In situations where food aid is already being delivered, the review of secondary data should pay close attention to the food aid and feeding programmes in place. Information on general food distribution is obviously very important in times of food insecurity. It is important to know:

- what the ration size and quality is, particularly for populations who are solely dependent on the ration
- what proportion of the population is receiving the ration compared to the size of the group targeted
- whether or not the distribution is equitable (ie, are any groups being excluded?)

The quantity of food being received needs to be reviewed in the light of the food security information and the likely requirements of the population. In situations *where people do not have other sources of food*, the recommended planning figure is 2,100kcals per person per day for food aid, although it is recommended that the requirements of the population are assessed in each context. Food aid in these situations should also meet protein, fat and micronutrient requirements.

If you need to check the nutritional content of ration profile, you can use nutval.xls, which is a spreadsheet on the CD-ROM attached to this manual. The analysis is based on the average population requirements recommended for planning.

A number of factors affect the nutritional requirements of a population. If these factors are very different from those assumed in the calculation of the planning figure then the planning figure should be adjusted accordingly. Factors assumed in the planning figure are as follows:

1. the demographic structure of the population is as shown in Table A2.2
2. the average weight of the population is 60kg for men and 52kg for women
3. people are only engaging in light physical activity
4. the ambient temperature is 20°C or more and people have adequate shelter and clothing
5. there is not a high rate of malnutrition or disease.

Table A2.2   Demographic structure of a typical population in the developing world

Group	Percentage of population
0–4 years	12
5–9 years	12
10–14 years	11
15–19 years	10
20–59 years	49
60+ years	7
Pregnant	2.5
Breastfeeding	2.5
Male/female ratio	51/49

If these assumptions are not true and you suspect the ration may be inadequate you should estimate how the planning figure should be adjusted using guidance in UNHCR/Unicef/WFP/WHO (2002) *Food and Nutrition Needs in Emergencies*, found on the CD-ROM attached to this manual.

If your secondary analysis of endemic micronutrient deficiencies has shown that rates of anaemia, iodine deficiency disorder (IDD) or vitamin A deficiency are high (see subsection A2.1.1) then it is important to assess whether measures are in place to prevent these deficiencies from becoming any more widespread. This involves finding out whether any salt distributed with the food ration is iodised and whether vitamin A or iron supplementation is taking place (see subsection A2.1.4 for more on this point).

Selective feeding programmes

Information on the existence of, access to and normal functioning of feeding centres should also be reviewed. Routine data gathered at supplementary and therapeutic feeding centres can help you to understand the wider nutritional environment. Therefore, you should try to obtain reports on these types of interventions from other agencies during the secondary data collection phase. Conclusions should always be drawn carefully and you should take into account as much information as possible.

It is useful to get information on the coverage of the programme (see Part F for a detailed description of how to assess coverage) as this will indicate the proportion of the target population being reached. An increase in admission rates into a feeding centre may be indicative of a decline in the food security situation or may be due to a disease outbreak. Either may be seasonally typical. Admission rates should always be examined in the light of other factors such as whether the coverage of the feeding centres has changed. For example, admissions appeared to rise in Save the Children feeding centres in Huambo, Angola in September 2000, but Médecins Sans Frontières (MSF) had closed two centres at that time which may have accounted for the increase in admissions to Save the Children centres.

Feeding centre readmission rates are a good indicator of how well the family is coping. A readmission is usually defined as a child who is admitted into a feeding programme within three months of exiting that same programme. Children are at risk of being readmitted if their family cannot afford to ensure that the nutritional needs of the child are met following nutritional rehabilitation in a feeding programme.

If the age profile of children admitted changes – eg, the proportion of children over five increases – this may be indicative of a change in the food or disease environment. Young children (under three years) are most vulnerable to infectious disease, so a high proportion of children in this age category is likely to reflect high rates of infection. Large proportions of older children, particularly children over five years, may be more indicative of a food security problem.

Wet feeding programmes for moderately malnourished children usually rely on the family providing some food in order for the child to meet their calorific requirements for catch-up growth. Dry rations usually allow for some food to be shared with other household members. If the household has a very high food insecurity and cannot access enough food to feed the other household members, either the normal allocation of food for the child admitted to the feeding centre is diverted to other children (in the case of wet feeding) or the dry ration is shared among all family members, thereby reducing the amount given to the child registered on the feeding programme. Both of these scenarios mean that the child will recover slowly, daily weight gain will be low and length of stay will be long. These indicators in a supplementary feeding centre can help us assess whether the child is receiving adequate food at home. Slow rates of weight gain may also result if underlying disease is not adequately identified and treated.

A2.1.4 Public health information

Reviewing information on health status is described in subsection A2.1.2. To review the public health situation you will require information on health services and the risk of disease.

Information on the health services currently available to the population is useful (see Section A1.4). This should include basic questions about whether or not there is a functioning health system, ie, the presence of trained and regularly paid health workers, systems of referral and access to essential drugs. Of particular interest is the vaccination status of the population, especially whether they have been vaccinated against measles. Vitamin A is also commonly given with measles vaccination and can be an important intervention when rates of infection are high. Review of secondary information should also try to establish whether there has been a recent vitamin A supplement distribution.

Insufficient water provision, in terms of both quantity and quality, increases the risk of diarrhoeal diseases and other water-borne diseases. Water is an important consideration for all populations, although the consequences of poor sanitation and hygiene in crowded camps for displaced people may be worse as they can lead to epidemics of cholera, etc. Assessment of sanitation facilities (access to and number of latrines) and practices (collection and disposal of solid waste) is very important in a camp situation. This information is less critical in a settled rural population. In places where people pay for water, prices can sharply increase during a drought, particularly in urban areas and dry areas. This results in people buying less water. Time spent on water collection influences water quality and time available for child care.

You should seek to answer the following questions relevant to health information in your review of the secondary data:

Basic health services
- What is the estimated measles vaccination coverage of the affected population?
- Is vitamin A routinely given with measles vaccination? What is the estimated vitamin A supplement coverage?
- What is the structure of the health system in the area?
- Are health facilities accessible and functioning?
- What is the level of BCG vaccination coverage?
- What is the availability of medication in other places (pharmacies, markets, etc)?
- How often is the population using the health services?
- What nutrition intervention or community-based support (eg, home-based

care for PLWH/A) was in place before the current emergency, or has been put in place since?

Public health environment
- Is there or will there be a significant decline in ambient temperature likely to affect the prevalence of ARI?
- Have people been in water or wet clothes for long periods of time?
- Is the water supply adequate (quantity, quality) or has it changed from normal?
- Are people buying water? Has the price changed?
- What is the distance to, and time of queuing at, the water point?
- Are people living in overcrowded conditions?

In displaced populations
- How many people are there per latrine?
- Have people moved from a non-endemic malarial zone to an endemic zone?

A2.1.5 Information on the social and care environment

In an emergency nutrition assessment we are primarily concerned with changes in the care environment which result from the emergency. Inappropriate caring practices present before the emergency take a long time to change and are best tackled through a development programme. You should therefore seek to answer the following questions in your review of the secondary data:

- Has there been a change in work patterns due to migration, displacement or armed conflict which means that roles and responsibilities in the household have changed?
- Is there a change in the normal composition of households and what is the cause of this? What is the dependency ratio?[4]
- Are there large numbers of separated children?
- Has the normal care environment been disrupted (for example, through displacement) affecting access to secondary carers, access to foods for children, access to water?
- What are the normal infant feeding practices? Are mothers bottle feeding their babies or using manufactured complementary foods? If so, is there an infrastructure that can support safe bottle feeding?
- Is there evidence of donations of baby foods and milks, bottles and teats or requests for donations?

---

[4] The dependency ratio is the ratio of active adults to dependants. The specific definition of an active adult should be defined locally. The effective dependency ratio is calculated differently and includes ill adults as dependants.

- In pastoral communities, have herds been away from young children for long? Has access to milk changed from normal?
- Has HIV/AIDS affected caring practices at household level, ie, has the burden of care increased?

Specific groups will be at a higher nutritional risk and should be identified in order to set priorities. Your review of secondary data should identify, where possible, specific groups of the population that face nutritional risk. Groups at potentially high risk include:

- the physiologically vulnerable, including children under five years (particularly those aged 6–24 months), pregnant and lactating women, adolescent girls, older and/or disabled people and the chronically ill, including people living with HIV/AIDS. These groups have special nutritional requirements (either in terms of quantity or quality) which may not be met during an emergency. As seen in Table A2.2 the extra nutrition needs of different age groups are taken into account in the average population planning figures for food aid. Food aid, however, is often in reality of inadequate quantity to meet the needs of these groups
- people discriminated against or marginalised, including female-headed households, disabled people, older people, orphans and unaccompanied children may find it difficult to access normal services and so may need extra assistance. Particular ethnic, religious, political or social groups can be marginalised by authorities and their access to basic services and/or food may be restricted.

The term vulnerable should not be used to mean the same thing as need, nor should it be regarded as an absolute status (ie, it is not true that female-headed households are always vulnerable). Rather it should be used to denote risk of malnutrition. Those who are vulnerable to malnutrition will vary from place to place and should be identified during the assessment rather than assumed.

A2.1.6 Basic causes of malnutrition

In your review of the basic causes of malnutrition you are primarily concerned with defining the shock(s) which characterises the emergency and then looking at how this shock leads to the underlying causes you have identified in your review. The following questions should be addressed:

- *What is the cause of the crisis?* It is important to know the cause of the crisis – whether it is man-made (war, political instability, economic, etc) or a natural disaster (drought, flooding, earthquake, pests, livestock or human epidemics, etc). Alternatively, the crisis may have been caused by a combination of man-made and natural disasters. You should find out how long the shock has been affecting the population? Have there been repeated shocks? Why has the shock occurred?

- *How secure is the population?* You need to know where the insecurity is concentrated, how fast the situation is changing and how the insecurity is manifesting itself. Have people been displaced? Have people's homes been burnt? Has people's land been mined or water sources bombed? Have family members and communities been separated? How are armed groups establishing their power? Which groups are the most powerful and which are the least powerful?

- *What is the environment like?* If people have been displaced, it is important to understand the environment in which they are now located and how different it is from the place where they were living. Do they have social connections in the new place? Are people likely to be experiencing cold or stress? Is the disease environment different in the new place? How far is the new place and how did they get there? The area from which a displaced population originates will affect their ability to cope in a new environment. For example, rural people may find it hard to cope in an urban environment and vice versa. Resident populations are often put under stress and destabilised when a displaced population arrives. They may also be in need and should not be forgotten when planning a response to a crisis. The relationship between the two populations will depend on kinship, ratio of displaced to resident, the economic situation and the residents' degree of food security. Population displacement should not be confused with temporary migration, which may be part of normal coping strategies.

- *How many people are affected?* You are specifically interested in the number of people affected in the area from which you will be sampling for the anthropometric and mortality surveys. Situation reports may include figures for a bigger area. Population figures are essential for planning any intervention.

A2.2 Sources of secondary information

There are many sources of secondary information, the majority of which can be explored before starting any field work for the assessment. Figure A2.2 shows the possible sources of information for each group of causes. In addition Appendix S1 lists useful websites for secondary information.

Figure A2.2 Sources of secondary information on the causes of malnutrition

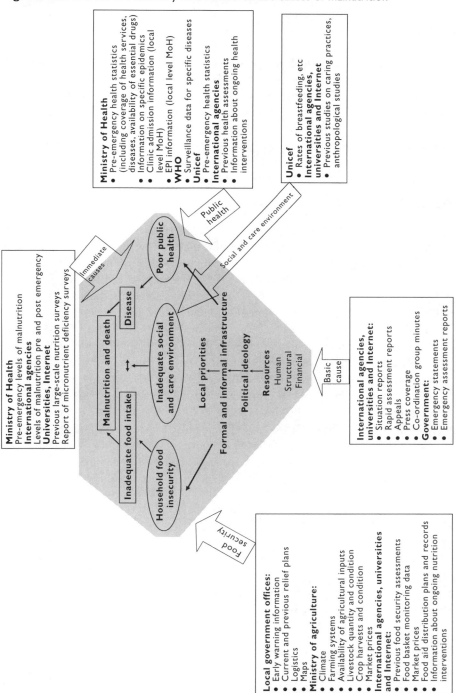

A2.3 Checking the accuracy and relevance of secondary information

Before deciding whether the secondary data you have reviewed can be used in the causal analysis you need to check the quality of the information you have found. You need to identify the information which appears to be accurate and relevant. It is possible that the information is accurate but *not* relevant – that is, if it is out of date or if it applies to a different population than the one you are considering. It is also possible that it is *not* accurate even though it could be relevant – that is, it is biased or likely to be wrong judging by the methods used for data collection. The worst scenario would be if it was neither accurate nor relevant.

A2.3.1 Out-of-date information

Some sources of secondary information may be out of date. This can mean that the data is just too old and therefore no longer relevant. Population data is the type of information that can go out of date very rapidly. Make sure you check several sources for information on population statistics. The most recent national level census is often five to ten years out of date. Displacement may completely change the location of entire communities.

Out-of-date information may also be a problem for food security assessments. You need to consider whether or not the conditions described in the report are still the same. Market price data can quickly be outdated in situations with hyperinflation. Crop conditions can change rapidly after rainfall. When you are considering secondary sources of information, like food security reports, you also need to remember that history does not necessarily repeat itself. Often, an attempt is made in an HEA report to predict the impact of a shock on the population's food security. However, if a population has faced more than one shock, or even a slightly different shock, the prediction may no longer be relevant.

Secondary information may also be irrelevant if it describes what is happening in a different season. Seasonality affects all the three underlying causes of malnutrition (see Section A1.6). This means that you need to be sure if, for example, you have a report about the incidence of malaria in a given area, that the report is for the relevant season. However, even if the information is not relevant to understanding the current situation, it could be useful when you are making recommendations concerning the future and judging how quickly the situation will get better or worse.

A2.3.2 Representativeness

You must make sure that the secondary information is representative of the whole population that you want to survey. In some cases, you may have information that only covers a certain section of the population: if this is so then you need to think about whether you can apply the conclusions of the data to the rest of the survey population, or whether you need to collect more information on the other groups.

Some examples of information which may not be relevant:

- National statistics on rates of breastfeeding may only have been gathered from parts of the country which were readily accessible for a national survey and may exclude the population of interest.
- A local health NGO may be working in one part of a district you are going to survey. The NGO has health information on this area but not the other parts of the district. Be careful not to extrapolate this data to the whole district unless you are sure that the health conditions are similar.
- Food security information may apply to a food economy zone whereas a nutrition assessment may be being conducted according to administrative boundaries. This means that you need to check the relevance of the food security information to the entire area being assessed.

A2.3.3 Biased and inaccurate information

You should be aware that secondary information can be biased. Bias is often difficult to detect. Information can be biased by the ideology or technical leanings of the data reporter, and it is difficult to detect bias unless you have some knowledge of why the information was collected.

Examples of biased information

- A sector-specific assessment may not take into account needs in other areas. For example, a water and sanitation assessment may not take into account the role which water can play in determining food security.
- Some sources may have a vested interest in providing biased population information. For example, authorities may want to exaggerate the number of people in a district in order to obtain more food aid. Alternatively, in some situations authorities may deliberately provide low estimates of minority population groups.

Bias can also be introduced through the methods used. Bias from using poor sampling techniques is discussed in detail for anthropometric and mortality surveys in Chapters B2 and C2. For example, a mortality survey which only surveys households with children under the age of five is biased as it may exclude households whose last-born child recently died. Qualitative assessments which only consider the views of men, or only consider the views of elders may also be biased or inaccurate in their conclusions (see Section A4.3 for more on this point).

Inaccurate information is a common problem, and it can arise for a number of reasons. The information could be fabricated or the wrong conclusions could be drawn from the information found. Generalising from anecdotes can be particularly misleading.

Examples of inaccurate information

- Routine health statistics may be fabricated in order to complete the forms at health centre level.
- Population statistics may be entirely made up. For example, it may be in the interests of an armed group controlling an area to state that everyone had fled their villages and no one was left.
- Comments about the behaviour of the affected population may be generalised. 'The male population is largely addicted to alcohol' – a conclusion drawn after the reporter saw a group of drunk men.
- A report could conclude that the population is receiving too much food aid because food aid was seen being sold on the market. In fact, people may be selling the food aid in order to buy soap or other essential items and cutting back on some of their consumption of food as a consequence.

A2.4 Recording your review of secondary information

As you conduct the review you should take notes on a page with two columns. The first column should note down the key points related to the causes of malnutrition (as identified in Section A2.1). In the second column, you should note any points concerning the relevance and accuracy of the report. An example of the output at the end of the secondary review of causes of malnutrition in Masisi, Democratic Republic of Congo is shown in Figure A2.3.

Figure A2.3 Example: Notes resulting from review of secondary data

Masisi is a territory in the east of North Kivu province at an altitude between 1,460m (bordering lake Kivu and near Goma) and 2,500m. The area suffered from inter-ethnic conflict between 1993 and 1999 and hosts many displaced people. Since security improved, many people have returned from Rwanda.

NGO mortality survey June 2001 • Results: Under-5 mortality rate (U5MR) 3/10,000/day.	Retrospective methodology on mortality unclear, potentially biased because the recall period was unusually long (12 months rather than the standard 3 months).
Save the Children HEA assessment April 2000 and update 2003 • Masisi household economy zone is the plateaux area, which is considered more vulnerable to food insecurity than other parts of the territory. • Main crops grown include beans, sweet potatoes, Irish potatoes, maize, sorghum and bananas. • Other economic activities include brewing, charcoal production and sale of firewood. Better-off households also involved in petty trade. • Lean period is September–November • Overall food security has improved over time, but there seems to be an increasing equity gap, while the 'poor' make up a smaller percentage of the population. • The causes of food insecurity are the influx of returnees, insecurity, reduction in land holding size, lack of access to markets, few income-generating activities or alternatives to agriculture.	Data is internally consistent, processed, not raw, includes analysis. Time constraints (3 days) for follow-up report. Limited analysis.
Routine health statistics **Masisi health zone 2001** • Mortality rate is highest April–July, which corresponds with the start of the rainy season. • Low utilisation rate of health centres.	Unclear how the clinic utilisation rate was calculated – not internally consistent. No information is provided on incidence of common diseases.

Summary

In order to conduct a review of secondary data, you need to try to answer key questions about the level of malnutrition before the emergency and the causes of malnutrition (immediate, underlying and basic, before and after the emergency). The shock should be considered a possible basic cause.

- Check the quality of your secondary data in relation to its accuracy and relevance.
- Record the results of your review carefully in preparation for constructing the pre-assessment causal pathway.

Chapter A3
Completing the pre-assessment causal framework

A3.1 Constructing the framework

After reviewing the secondary information, you should know something about the situation of the population that has been affected by the emergency with respect to the immediate, underlying and basic causes of malnutrition. You should also have information on the extent of malnutrition prior to the current emergency.

Once you have checked the secondary information (see Section A2.3) you need to discard the information which is useless – that is, information which is inaccurate or not relevant enough or too biased. You then need to construct the pre-assessment causal framework. To do this you should undertake three tasks.

1. Write out a flipchart showing the causes and extent of malnutrition prior to the emergency. You may find it easier to write each of the causes on a small card or sticky note so that they can be moved around.
2. Write out a flipchart showing the causes of malnutrition following the emergency. Some of these causes will be the same as for 1) above, others will be new, as a result of the emergency. Causes of malnutrition which exist as a consequence of the emergency may be being partially (or fully) addressed by existing relief operations. It is therefore very important to take these into account in the framework. Included in the basic causes should be a description of the shock itself (see Figure A3.1).
3. Seasonal variation in the causes should be captured. This should include, where possible, information for the months which follow the assessment so that later judgements can be made on whether the situation is likely to get better or worse. It may be easier to plot these changes on a seasonal calendar (see also subsection A4.4.5).

The completion of flipcharts should be a team exercise. Points which are not agreed by all members or for which data is possibly biased or inaccurate should be identified with a question mark.

A3.2 Identifying gaps, inconsistencies and issues needing validation

Your next step is to review your pre-assessment causal framework and identify the gaps in your understanding, which pieces of information you need to validate in the assessment and which information needs further cross-checking during the assessment.

It is best to look at the framework as a team. Ideally, you will have someone who knows the survey area with you when you are discussing the findings from the secondary sources. One useful way to approach the problem is suggested below.

- Working together as a team, agree on what information you are missing. It might help to cross-check the information you have with the lists of questions in Section A2.1.
- Work out which pieces of secondary information you are unsure about. Do this by trying to see that the whole 'story' makes sense. Are there any anomalies or inconsistencies? Do the different sources agree with each other?
- Identify the information which is so important that, even if you already have that information, you would like to gather it again during the assessment. An example could be measles vaccination and vitamin A supplementation coverage data: this is very easily gathered as part of the anthropometric survey and is so important for informing recommendations that it is probably worth always collecting it as primary data during the assessment.
- On a new flipchart, make a list of information you are missing. Start by grouping together the different types of missing information (health, food security, basic causes, etc) (see Figure A3.1).

A3.3 Gaps which always exist

At this stage in the assessment there will always be two important gaps in the information which you need. These are:

- information about the community's perceived needs
- information about the operational feasibility of any interventions you propose.

Chapter A4 suggests ways of gathering this information. At this stage you should brainstorm, on the basis of the causal framework, about what interventions could address the causes of malnutrition you have identified so far. This will help you to narrow down your questions on operational feasibility.

Figure A3.1 Example of a pre-assessment causal framework, from Masisi, Democratic Republic of Congo, after emergency

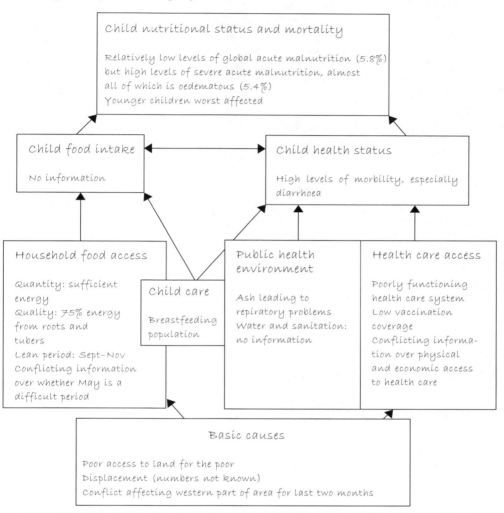

Child nutritional status and mortality

Relatively low levels of global acute malnutrition (5.8%) but high levels of severe acute malnutrition, almost all of which is oedematous (5.4%)
Younger children worst affected

Child food intake

No information

Child health status

High levels of morbility, especially diarrhoea

Household food access

Quantity: sufficient energy
Quality: 75% energy from roots and tubers
Lean period: Sept–Nov
Conflicting information over whether May is a difficult period

Child care

Breastfeeding population

Public health environment

Ash leading to repiratory problems
Water and sanitation: no information

Health care access

Poorly functioning health care system
Low vaccination coverage
Conflicting information over physical and economic access to health care

Basic causes

Poor access to land for the poor
Displacement (numbers not known)
Conflict affecting western part of area for last two months

Gaps identified

- Immediate causes: What are the morbidity patterns? Which period of the year carries the greatest nutritional risk: May or September–November?
- Care: Have child care practices have been disrupted by displacement?
- Food security: How bad is the lean period in terms of diet? Are there problems with preparation of tubers?
- Public health: What is the water and sanitation situation? How far are people from health facilities?
- Need better quality mortality data

Summary

In developing a pre-assessment causal pathway you need to do the following:

- Discard information from the secondary review which is not usable.
- Produce two flipcharts of the causes identified: one for before the emergency and one for after. Capture seasonal variation in the causes of malnutrition, ideally on a seasonal calendar.
- Identify gaps, inconsistencies and issues needing cross-checking and validation. It is useful to always identify measles vaccination and vitamin A supplement coverage as an issue requiring validation.
- Remember that you will always have gaps in information on the community's perceived needs and the operational feasibility of prospective interventions.
- Brainstorm on possible ideas for intervention to help limit the primary data collection required on investigating operational feasibility.

Chapter A4
Collecting primary information on causes of malnutrition

A4.1 How to develop a primary data collection plan

This chapter will help you decide how to collect primary information on the causes of malnutrition and, therefore, how to develop your data collection plan. You need to begin with the list of gaps that need to be filled (see Sections A3.2 and A3.3). Before starting the primary data collection you need to have made the following decisions:

1. Is there any information which could be gathered through secondary data available at field level? eg, health statistics from local health posts, population statistics, food aid distribution reports.
   If so, who will be responsible for obtaining this?
   See Section A2.2 for sources of secondary information.

2. Will any information be gathered through a household questionnaire?
   If so, will the questionnaire be part of the anthropometric or mortality survey?
   Subsection A4.2.1 discusses how you can decide between quantitative and qualitative techniques. Section A4.5 will help you decide which specific information could be collected through a household questionnaire.

3. What information will be gathered through qualitative techniques?

   • How will the information be collected (a key informant interview, focus group discussion, direct observation, a market survey, a calendar)?
   • Who should collect the information?
   • Which key informants should be used?
   • What questions should be posed?

Subsection A4.2.1 discusses how you can decide between quantitative and qualitative techniques. Section A4.3 describes the principles of qualitative data collection and Section A4.4 describes the different qualitative techniques that can be used. Section A4.5 will help you decide which specific information is best collected through qualitative techniques.

Remember that when you make these decisions you need to keep in mind the logistical and time constraints which you may face in the data collection.

A4.2 Deciding the methods to use

A4.2.1 Quantitative or qualitative?

Information on causes of malnutrition in a nutrition assessment is usually best gathered through qualitative methods. This is because the process needs to be iterative. This means that you will be testing out theories or assumptions and then, as you go, revising your questions based on the answers you are getting. The gaps in understanding identified when compiling the pre-assessment causal framework are unlikely to fit into neat questions which could be analysed as part of a quantitative survey.

If we return to the example in Section A3.2, the first gap was a lack of understanding of the impact of displacement on caring practices. It would be difficult and, more importantly, very limiting to, for example, ask about rates of breastfeeding among the mothers interviewed during the anthropometric assessment. First, this would not tell us anything about the effect of displacement; and second, care practices are much more far-reaching than breastfeeding. Instead, we could consider doing the following, through the use of qualitative techniques:

• Talk to groups of displaced women with young children to ask them about how far they have come from their homes, how they have coped with breastfeeding, what they are managing to provide in terms of complementary foods, and how this has changed since they were at home.
• Talk to village leaders about whether there are any children separated during the displacement.
• Visit a feeding centre or clinic to find out if there has been an increase in admissions of infants.
• Talk to older displaced people to find out what happened to elderly people during the displacement.
• Develop a time calendar with a groups of displaced and host community women to determine how much time they have available for child care.

This would allow us to investigate a broad range of possible answers to the question. If it becomes clear quickly that most people have not been displaced far from home and their caring practices have not altered very much, this line of enquiry could be stopped and collection of information on other areas prioritised.

In some instances, however, the information required could usefully be gathered in a quantitative survey. Household questionnaires are used to obtain information at household level. Questionnaires can be added to either the anthropometric survey (where households with children aged 6–59 months are included in the sample) or the mortality survey (where all households are included). Information about the food security situation may be best obtained from all households, whereas questions on the health situation may be best asked in households where there are young children. A household questionnaire gives a broad picture of what is happening, without the bias introduced by questioning only special-interest groups.

Example A4.1

Imagine you want to know who is receiving food aid in the survey population. If you ask community leaders or government officials, they may answer that everyone is receiving food aid equally. If you ask people at household level you can check this, and be sure that no particular group is being excluded.

There is *no standard* household questionnaire for an emergency nutrition assessment. In many situations there is no need for a household questionnaire at all. For example, if you think that all households are living in a very similar way, then it would save time to conduct only key informant interviews.

If you decide to collect information through a questionnaire, you need to keep in mind the analysis of the data. For example, if you ask the question 'Do you have any food stocks?', and the results show that 30% of households do have food stocks, how do you interpret this information? It would only be worth asking this question if you knew, from your food security assessment, that in a normal year, and at the time of the survey, 50% of households should have stocks and you knew the implications of reduced stocks on household access to food.

A4.2.2 Triangulation

Triangulation is a technique used to enhance the validity of the data collection process. Triangulation means taking information about the same issue from a variety of sources and comparing it to see if the findings are the same or different. If they are different, then either more sources should be sought to determine the correct conclusion or data suspected of being biased or inaccurate should be discarded.

There are two types of triangulation:

1) triangulation by comparing information gathered through different methods, eg, comparing morbidity information gathered through interviewing Ministry of Health (MoH) staff and morbidity information gathered through a questionnaire added to the anthropometric survey

2) triangulation by comparing information gathered through the same technique but by different observers, eg, comparing observations on

household access to water made by two different people on your assessment team.

While triangulation is essentially done at the time of analysis (and is dealt with primarily in Chapter A5), it is important when deciding your methods to understand its importance for ensuring the validity of your findings. When you are deciding how you will collect primary data on the causes of malnutrition, it may be a good idea to collect some information through a questionnaire and some through using qualitative techniques, or to ensure that several people on the survey team are asking the same questions in key informant interviews.

A4.3 Principles of qualitative data collection

It is important to recognise that in gathering qualitative information you are not trying to construct a statistically representative sample. Within the constraints of time, cost and access, your aim is to compile a description of the nutrition situation that is sufficient to allow you to understand the situation and make reasonable recommendations. Your confidence in the results of the interviews should be based on the consistency of the information received.

Measures need to be in place to ensure the quality of the data collection and avoid bias.

A4.3.1 Selection of locations

There are no fixed rules about how you select locations for your investigation. In practice, this is always a trade-off between logistics, capacity to inform and discuss options with people living in the location, time, and your desire to visit as many places as possible. You will usually be gathering this information at the same time as the anthropometric and mortality surveys, which means you may be restricted to visiting only the clusters or locations which are selected for sampling.

Your choice of locations will depend on the issues you want to investigate. You need to choose locations where you can access the groups of people about which you have questions. For example, if you have a question about how displaced people are coping and what the impact of their arrival is on the host population, it would make sense to visit clusters or locations where you know displaced people are.

If you want to investigate a cause of malnutrition which you suspect may not be uniform across the area you could decide to visit locations where you expect its impact to vary in order to test your assumptions. For example, if you think that a crop pest may be a particularly important cause of malnutrition but you suspect that the areas near the river were least affected because they tend to grow fewer crops, you could visit a location in the highly cropped area and a location by the river and perhaps a location in between. This would allow you to investigate your assumptions.

Always bear in mind that you are trying to develop an understanding of the causes as they affect most people in the area. That does not prevent you from looking at the situation of specific vulnerable groups but it would be a mistake to investigate only a group that you think is worst affected without getting an understanding of whether their circumstances were more broadly applicable.

A4.3.2 Who you should talk to

As with deciding where you should go, you should also think carefully about who you should talk to, again depending on the information you require. It's not very useful to talk to men about breastfeeding practices or to talk to farmers about fishing yields. You need to keep in mind that the groups you may wish to talk to may only feel comfortable to discuss the issues if they are with other people in a similar situation. For example, it may be difficult for poor women to discuss their hygiene practices in front of better-off women. You may also need to specifically request to meet groups of people who are not normally put forward to have discussions with outsiders – eg, children, disabled people, the destitute or the chronically ill. You may also need to adapt your techniques when interviewing these groups.[1]

Remember that, while it is important to talk to several people or groups about the same question, it is also important that different investigators ask the question. When an investigator tries to find out information they will always influence the information which is received, so if several investigators are exploring the same question the risks of bias overall are reduced.

A4.3.3 Field testing

As with quantitative methods, qualitative methods that you plan to use should always be field tested in advance of data collection. This allows you to test the questions you plan to pose and identify areas where bias could be introduced. It also allows all the members of the team to practise using the methods to get the same information.

---

[1] For more information on talking to these groups, see Laws, S (2003) *Research for Development*, Save the Children and Sage.

A4.3.4 The importance of accurate recording

It is very important that you always keep good notes of your qualitative data collection. Because information is gathered through conversation and observation, it is easy to forget to document it carefully. You should take care to separate in your notes the information given to you and your interpretations of the interview or comments on how it went.

A4.4 Qualitative techniques

A4.4.1 Key informant interviews and focus group discussions

Semi-structured interviewing is a way of informally guiding a discussion to obtain information. The interviewer often has a checklist of key areas he or she wishes to learn about. The structure is flexible, to allow the interviewer to follow up points of interest and ask new questions that arise as the discussion continues. Semi-structured interviews are an extremely useful way of obtaining a lot of information relatively quickly. They are also a useful way to understand the different ways in which different groups (for example, different livelihood or wealth groups) are coping with the situation. Be clear in advance about when you want to know about people's experience as opposed to when you are asking for their opinion.

You should remember that your style will affect the quality of the information you receive. Your body language, dress and spoken language will all affect the respondents and how they perceive your questions. Ensure in advance that you adopt approaches that are likely to enhance rather than inhibit the collection of good-quality information.

It is useful when conducting these interviews to repeat back to the group or key informant your understanding of what they are saying. This gives them the opportunity to correct any misunderstanding and will strengthen your understanding. It may also give you an opportunity to clarify any queries.

Using an interpreter
An interpreter is used to translate, as accurately as possible the questions put by the interviewer, not to insert their own opinions. Always take time before the interview to discuss with the translator the techniques you will be using and the general topic of conversation. Ask for a literal translation, rather than their personal interpretation. Tell them that you would like to hear their impressions afterwards, but that during the interview you want to hear the interviewee's exact words. Wherever possible, try to work with the same interpreter throughout. A good interpreter is a partner, who knows how to manage a group properly and can steer you out of trouble if you ask an inappropriate question. The best

interpreters will quickly grasp the purpose and logic of the interview, and with practice, should be able to conduct interviews on their own. If an interpreter is really unsatisfactory find someone more suitable – it is impossible to conduct good fieldwork with inadequate translation.

A4.4.2 Direct observation

Direct observation, by looking and learning, is one of the best ways to cross-check what people are saying. For example, if stories of severe malnutrition and dead livestock are common, have you seen this, and if not why not? Direct observation involves looking at the environment, the condition of the harvest and livestock, the physical appearance of the population and their living conditions (household hygiene, etc). Observation can also provide information about social interactions and caring practices. Important places to visit and observe during assessments include markets, health centres, water sources and food distribution sites.

A4.4.3 Market price data

The objectives of market data collection are to:

- find out current cereal and livestock prices for comparison with other years
- estimate the availability of food in the market
- estimate the terms of trade.

The information should be collected from local and major markets and from traders, as the situation will vary. You should interview both traders and local people who are selling livestock or cereals in the market. You should ensure you always compare the same foods (eg, variety and origin).

When collecting the information it is important to take precautions against recording inflated prices. If people know that the information is going to be used for relief purposes, they may inflate the prices. Remember to take a standard local measure so that you can easily convert cereal prices per local measure into kilograms. It is also important to obtain information about where the grains or animals have come from. Prices of foods normally depend on the source, local availability, how far they've come, and road accessibility. If the area is normally self-sufficient, but currently dependent on imported grains, this could be a sign of a food crisis. Price comparisons should be made with prices recorded in previous years during the same season. When baseline data is not available you can interview traders for this information. Remember that you can cross-check data from market surveys with the Ministry of Agriculture (MoA) and key informants from the community.

Figure A4.1 Seasonal Calendar for Huambo city, Angola, September 2000

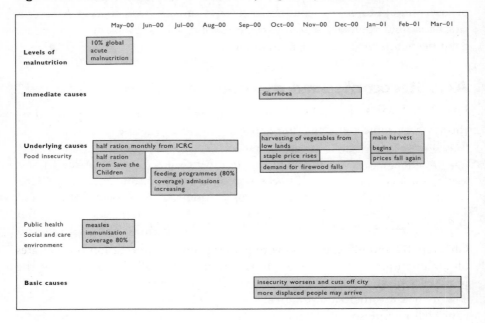

A4.4.5 Calendars

Seasonal calendars are a means of recording events during the year. They can be constructed in a number of ways, and before, during or after a visit to a community. We recommend developing a seasonal calendar before the fieldwork starts (see Section A3.1) and then revising it during the fieldwork.

Seasonal calendars can include any number of topics, such as harvest and planting times, sales of livestock, purchase of grain, movement to grazing lands, peak fishing times, sickness among children, etc. See Figure A4.1 for an example. The advantage of a seasonal calendar is that it presents visually a number of different activities that are carried out at the same time, enabling you to see the correlation between them. For instance, if peak labour requirements occur at the same time as planting and harvest, it is likely that smaller households will not be able to devote much time to their own plots. Because seasonal calendars reveal a range of possible interconnections, they can spark off interesting debates. Calendars can also take into account events which are likely to occur after the assessment, which will help later on in interpreting the severity of the findings from the anthropometric and mortality surveys (see Chapter D1).

Constructing a calendar in a village often works best with a group. The exercise works better if there is a mixture of people. Constructing time calendars over a 24-hour period with care givers can also be useful in helping understand the impact of the emergency on caring practices. This can show, for example, the amount of time a carer spent collecting fuel and therefore was separated from his or her young children, or standing in queues to receive assistance, or caring for sick household members. These observations can help with the development of recommendations for future programmes.

A4.5 Recommended methods for different types of information

In this section we will review how best to collect primary information on the causes of malnutrition and other factors (such as the community's perceived needs). Remember to refer back to Section A2.1 to find out the sort of information you need.

A4.5.1 Rates of malnutrition and mortality

Chapters B2 and C2 explain how to gather primary information on the rates of malnutrition and mortality. It is not usually realistic to measure the prevalence of micronutrient deficiency in an emergency nutrition assessment. This is because there are few field-friendly methods for assessment and the team will require specialist training. Subsection A2.1.3 describes information needed for determining risk of micronutrient deficiency. In a situation where a micronutrient deficiency outbreak is suspected – because of surveillance data or cases presenting at health centres – a specialist team for assessing the scale of the problem may be required.

A4.5.2 Immediate causes

Health status

Probably the best way to get information on morbidity is from MoH staff and through discussions with women or community leaders. They can tell you if there have been any outbreaks and what the major illnesses are at the time of the survey. It may be useful to plot a seasonal calendar of morbidity to compare the current situation with expected patterns – this will help you work out whether or not the situation is 'normal' for the time of year.

Good data on morbidity is difficult to obtain from questionnaires. Different people understand different things by diarrhoea or fever, so you have to use standardised case definitions; these can sometimes be difficult to formulate. Also, some symptoms (like diarrhoea and fever) are associated with more than one disease (like malaria and measles). A further problem is that we don't really know what the 'normal' level is for many of the symptoms. In other words, we don't know when there is an abnormally high incidence of diarrhoea or fever. This makes interpretation of morbidity data information very difficult. If we can't interpret the data then there is no point in collecting it (see also subsection A4.5.2).

Information on measles is an exception to this rule because mothers can nearly always recognise it and even one case is potentially dangerous. You should always therefore include a question about measles in your anthropometric survey, but make sure you find out what the appropriate local term for measles is. The WHO definition for a measles case is:

'Any person in whom a clinician suspects measles infection or any person with fever, and maculopapular rash (ie, non-vesicular), and cough, coryza (ie, runny nose) or conjunctivitis (ie, red eyes).'[2]

Questions about symptoms (usually diarrhoea, fever and cough/difficult breathing) can also be included, but only if there is a standard case definition commonly used in the country in which you are working and you know what is 'normal' for the area (see Table A4.1). For example, a common definition of diarrhoea for children over six months is three or more loose stools per day. Again, remember to make sure you get the right local name for a particular symptom. In general, the mother is asked whether or not the child has suffered from this symptom at any time during the past 14 days, although some agencies prefer to ask about the previous 24 hours only, to reduce recall error.

Table A4.1 Example of morbidity questions that might be added to an anthropometric questionnaire

Has (NAME of CHILD) had measles in the past two weeks?	Yes / No
Has (NAME of CHILD) had diarrhoea* in the past two weeks?	Yes / No
Has (NAME of CHILD) had a fever* in the past two weeks?	Yes / No
Has (NAME of CHILD) had a cough* or had difficulty breathing in the past two weeks?	Yes / No
Has (NAME of CHILD) suffered from any other symptom in the past two weeks?	Yes / No

* defined according to local case definition

Food intake

It is not advisable to gather information on an individual's food intake in a nutrition assessment primarily because this information is very difficult and time consuming to obtain (Gibson, 1990). In most instances, you just need to assume that if a household is food secure then household members

[2] See http://www.who.int/vaccines-surveillance/deseasedesc/RSS_measles.htm'RecCaseDef

will be consuming adequate quantities of food according to their needs. Conversely, if the household is food insecure, then you should assume that some, or all, members of the household will be consuming less than their requirements.

In some situations, where you have reason to suspect that feeding practices have changed because of the emergency you may need to look more closely into what children are being fed. However, this usually requires a fairly complex questionnaire and much more time. Detailed descriptions on how to collect and analyse information on young children's feeding practices can be found in Ruel and Arimond (2003) on the CD-ROM.

The identification of nutritionally vulnerable groups (see subsection A2.1.5) may provide information about who is finding it difficult to access food available within a household or indeed about individuals who are not in households. However, it will not usually be possible to measure the food intake of these groups.

A4.5.3 Food security information

Household food security is best assessed using qualitative methods. Save the Children usually collects food security information using the Household Economy Approach (see subsection A2.1.3). HEA gathers qualitative and quantitative information using qualitative methods, eg, focus group discussions. This approach assesses the population's food security at a baseline and then reviews the effects of the shock on current and future food security. Alternatively, another agency's qualitative assessment of household food security could be used. These should both be reviewed alongside other secondary data discussed in Chapter A2.

If a baseline assessment is available and it simply needs to be reviewed in the light of the current crisis, this can be conducted quite quickly by a specialist food security team. If, however, there is no baseline information available considerably more resources and time will be required. The collection of information needed for an HEA is not straightforward and takes time. It should only be undertaken by people who have been trained in the method.

If the household food security information is available then there is normally no need to collect new information on food security during your nutrition survey. You may, however, wish to cross-check information during the nutrition assessment or find out whether all the vulnerable groups identified in the secondary data review are adequately represented in the food security assessment. This is probably best done through qualitative techniques, although specific questions may be added to a household questionnaire. For example, if the food security assessment predicts that following the failure of the rains, milk access will continue to deteriorate for all wealth groups for the subsequent nine months, then the household questionnaires could ask a question about milk access in order to triangulate this information with the secondary information.

Similarly, market price data gathered during the assessment can help to validate secondary food security information. Household questionnaires can also be a useful means of assessing access to relief food by asking questions about receipt of ration, quantities received, frequency of distribution and access to distribution point. Feeding programme coverage is best obtained through a quantitative survey (see Part F).

It is very rare for there to be no food security information at all on the population. There may be circumstances where available information is very limited – eg, in an area that has previously been very insecure. Under these circumstances, which it is stressed are *not* ideal, it may be necessary to collect food security data during the nutrition assessment. You should only proceed with this if you have someone in your team who is familiar with working on food security information (see Part E for more information on nutrition assessment team composition).

Different types of food security information can be collected using different methods during a nutrition assessment. Some aspects can be incorporated into a household-level questionnaire, but other factors require in-depth discussion. Your main objective in collecting food security information during a nutrition assessment is to answer the questions described in subsection A2.1.3. Questions could be posed in a questionnaire on the following issues:

- access to specific nutrients – eg, protein foods (meat, fish, pulses, milk, blood)
- food purchases of key food items – like milk for pastoralists, groundnuts for maize-eating population
- household food stocks – eg, cereal grain
- absence of household members – due to labour migration, war, etc
- use of different types of coping strategies – firewood collection, water selling, large-scale slaughtering of animals, asset sales, unusual migration, etc.

Figure A4.2 provides examples of coping strategies as they become more destructive to livelihoods. It is impossible to provide a generic set of coping strategies which are damaging in all contexts. Thus, in an emergency prone context, it is likely to be more appropriate to determine the coping strategies normally used in emergency times and monitor their use over time. This approach is described in detail in Maxwell et al, 2003.

Many other aspects of food security are then best dealt with using qualitative approaches, including assessing the risk of micronutrient deficiency. This will include observation, mapping, construction of seasonal calendars and historical datelines, wealth ranking and proportional piling. Most important, however, are

Figure A4.2 Examples of progression from normal activity to unsustainable and damaging activity

Coping Strategies		
Sequential use	Examples of strategies	Characteristics
Reference *Normal activities*		• Typical seasonal exploitation of domestic resources & economic opportunities
STAGE I **Neutral coping strategies** (insurance mechanisms and coping strategies that are not damaging to livelihoods)	• Changes in cropping and planting practices • Sale of smallstock • Changes in diet (eg. switching to cheaper foods) • Collection of wild foods • Use of inter-household transfers and loans • Increased petty commodity production • Migration in search of employment • Sale of possessions (eg. jewelry)	• Risk-minimising • Loss-management • Low commitment of domestic resources
STAGE 2 **Destructive coping strategies** (Strategies that are damaging to nutritional status and livelihoods – particularly disposal of productive assets)	• Sale of livestock (eg, oxen) • Sale of agricultural tools • Sale or mortgaging of land • Credit from merchants and moneylenders • Reduction of current consumption levels	• High commitment of domestic resources • Unsustainable
STAGE 3 **Destitution**	• Distress migration	• Failure to cope

the key informant discussions with members of different livelihood and/or wealth groups. Always remember to seek out representatives of vulnerable groups for these discussions too. Other good sources of information on food security are MoA staff and local agricultural extension workers.

A4.5.4 Public health information

Information on measles vaccinations and vitamin A supplementation rates should always be collected during an anthropometric survey because of their relationship with mortality and malnutrition. Information about BCG scars can also usefully be collected during an anthropometric survey.

- In some countries measles vaccinations are given either during campaigns or during a routine expanded programme of immunisation (EPI). Children should be vaccinated for measles at nine months. You can tell whether or not a child has had a measles vaccination by examining her/his vaccination card, or by asking her/his carer to remember whether or not s/he has been vaccinated.
- When asking a mother about vitamin A supplementation, it is useful to bring a capsule with you. Show the mother the capsule and ask if her child has taken one of the capsules in the past six months (the capsules are normally distributed in conjunction with vaccination campaigns).
- BCG vaccinations are relatively easy to detect: look for a scar on the upper arm. The scar is normally on the right arm, but may be on the left, so check both.[3]

Table A4.2 Example of questions about measles, vitamin A supplementation and BCG vaccinations that can be added to an anthropometric questionnaire

Has (NAME of CHILD) been vaccinated for measles?	(1 = yes, confirmation with card) (2 = yes, no card but carer can confirm) (0 = not vaccinated)
Has (NAME of CHILD) received a vitamin A capsule in the past six months?	(Y = yes) (N = no) (DK = don't know)
Does (NAME of CHILD) have a BCG vaccination scar?	(Y = yes) (N = no)

It is useful to triangulate the information you collect on measles, vitamin A supplementation and BCG from the survey with information from interviews with the MoH.

Basic information about access to health services and whether or not they are functioning, etc is best sought from a mixture of observation and key informant interviews with MoH staff, women and community leaders. A detailed

---

[3] The scar has been described as a round, slightly depressed area with irregular edges, 4–7 mm in diameter. Occasionally it is raised a few millimetres above the skin as a result of fibrous tissue formation and is hard to the touch or healing may be accompanied by a retracted scar (PAHO, 1986).

description on how to assess water, hygiene and sanitation is provided in The Sphere Project handbook (2004), pages 89–92.

A4.5.5 Information on the social and care environment

In emergency nutrition assessments, household questionnaires are unlikely to be the best way to gather information on caring practices because it can take a long time to get the detailed information that you need.[4] Usually, it is more helpful to interview groups of mothers in key informant discussions to obtain information on caring practices. Remember that you are trying to find out if the emergency has resulted in any changes in caring practices which would negatively affect malnutrition.

Another reason that household questionnaires are not normally the best way to get information on caring practices is because of the sample size needed to get reliable information. The most common inappropriate caring practices take place in infancy (for example, non-exclusive breastfeeding and poor complementary feeding). The standard anthropometric survey focuses on children 6–59 months old and so there will only be a limited number of children aged 6–23 months; children under six months are excluded. It is therefore likely that the sample size for children aged 6–23 months would not be big enough to obtain statistically meaningful results. Therefore, if there is specific concern that infant feeding practices have changed as a consequence of the emergency or are particularly dangerous, an infant feeding survey should be conducted (see Ruel and Arimond, 2003, on CD-ROM).

It is possible to add questions about the dependency ratio to the mortality survey questionnaire. This will involve asking about the age of household members and (if you are calculating the effective dependency ratio – see subsection A2.1.5) whether any of them are chronically ill. It could also involve asking who the household head is to find out whether the age or sex of the household head is associated with particularly high dependency ratios.

As indicated in subsection A2.1.5, information on the groups facing nutritional risk should be gathered. This is sometimes done by asking about a specific characteristic in a questionnaire (eg, female-headed household, if the child is an orphan, if the household is made up of internally displaced persons (IDPs). This information is gathered with a view to then analysing the prevalence of malnutrition in these different population subgroups. This is only a good idea if your population subgroups are large (ie, you end up with a large sample from each subgroup), otherwise there will be very little statistical power to draw conclusions (see example A4.4).

---

[4] Information on how to collect data on child-caring practices is described in detail in Ruel and Arimond (2003).

The remaining information required to understand the impact of the shock on the social and care environment can probably best be obtained through qualitative methods including focus group discussions and observation.

Example A4.4
A survey conducted in Zimbabwe in 2004 showed that 8.5% of children in the sample were orphans. Levels of malnutrition among the 79 children who had lost their father appeared to be similar to overall rates but of the three children who had lost their mother one was malnourished, suggesting a high rate of malnutrition. The numbers of children in this group were, however, far too small to draw any conclusions.

A4.5.6 Information on basic causes

Qualitative techniques are best used to gather any necessary information about the shock and the numbers of affected people. Observation is a useful technique to cross-check information gained through focus group discussion and key informant interview: eg, population figures could be cross-checked roughly by door-counting in a community, or the impact of a drought on the harvest could be cross-checked by looking at the crop in the fields or looking at people's grain stores. Up-to-date information on the security situation is often best gained through discussion at local level rather than through secondary sources.

A4.5.7 Community's perceived needs

Seeking the views of the community on their needs is a very important part of the assessment process. They may have very clear ideas about the nature of the problem and its solution, and it is important that recommendations ultimately made in the nutrition assessment take these views into account. Some communities may be totally opposed to targeting food aid. For example, in parts of southern Sudan, social obligations to redistribute food to those who need it exist within the community. People in communities may perceive their needs differently from outsiders. In many situations a large proportion of a population face no risk of starvation and are chiefly preoccupied with preserving their assets and securing their means of subsistence in the long term, eg, minimising current consumption to avoid selling livestock or other productive assets, while outsiders may place more emphasis on preventing starvation. Some communities may perceive those in greatest need to be those who are socially vulnerable – eg, the old, widows, orphans, etc – and may not agree with interventions targeted according to economic and physiological vulnerability. You need to find out about systems like this if you are going to plan a useful intervention (see Table A4.3).

Table A4.3 Summary of information on the community's perceived needs required in an emergency nutrition assessment

Information required	How / where to obtain the information
• What are the community's immediate concerns and priorities for intervention? • How do they regard the situation compared with other crisis episodes? • What do they think is the best mechanism for relief distribution, if it is required? • Who does the community think is most vulnerable? • What capacity for implementation of the relief operation already exists in the community?	• Key informant interviews and focus group discussions with different population groups — rich/poor, agriculturalists/pastoralists, men/women

In addition, it is important that recommendations build on existing capacities in the community rather than assuming that assistance has to be provided entirely by outsiders. This involves finding out, for example, who has been trained in the community in relevant activities, what networks for delivering assistance could be tapped into, and which systems of local authority are most effective for delivery of assistance.

A4.5.8 Information on operational feasibility

During the assessment itself, it will not be possible to determine the detailed operational feasibility of potential interventions to treat or prevent malnutrition. A feasibility assessment is a necessary prerequisite for any decision to intervene and cannot be appropriately incorporated into an assessment of needs. However, it is important that recommendations are not wildly unfeasible, and therefore some basic information should be collected using qualitative techniques.

Access
This information is necessary to determine strategies, programme design and the scale of the intervention. Information on the main constraints met by the local community and by other agencies working in the area (security, environmental, logistical) is required. The information must consider access to the population in need – eg, presence and condition of roads, availability of an airstrip, or alternative modes of transport for local and regional transport capacity.

Resources and storage

When planning the procurement of any substance (food, medicine) it is necessary to know what is already available. The presence or absence of skilled personnel at local level is important when designing programmes. Are trained personnel available to run supplementary feeding programmes and therapeutic feeding programmes? Lists of possible locations (health facilities, buildings, etc) where feeding or storage centres could be implemented are important for planning.

Summary

In developing a plan for collecting primary data on the causes of malnutrition, the following issues need to be considered:

- Is there more information which could be gathered from secondary sources at field level?
- Is primary information best gathered through quantitative or qualitative techniques? In most instances, qualitative techniques will provide the most appropriate method. Methods should be chosen with the aim of triangulating information from a number of sources.
- When qualitative methods are used, specific techniques should be carefully chosen and strategies developed to minimise bias.

Chapter A5
Analysing the data and revising the causal framework

A5.1 How the information should be analysed

A5.1.1 Analysis during the data collection period

You should start analysing the causal data during the data collection period. Make sure you learn as you go while you are conducting the fieldwork. If possible, you should have a team debriefing session every night so that you can discuss your findings. During these sessions you should return to the pre-assessment causal framework and seasonal calendar and start to revise them on the basis of the information you are receiving. At these sessions you should be asking the team the following questions:

- Do we have any new information on the causes of malnutrition?
- Does this information confirm/fit in with the information we already have on the causal framework and seasonal calendar? Do the differences in information represent the experience of different parts of the population? If not, what should we do to find out which information is correct?
- Do the causes link together? Are there linkages between the basic, underlying and immediate causes?
- Are there any reasons to suspect that any of the information we have is biased? How could we obtain unbiased information on this issue?
- Which information has only come from one source and needs to be validated with other sources?
- What information do we still need to obtain?

The process of analysing data on the causes of malnutrition should be iterative. You need to constantly refine analysis as new pieces of information come to light.

A5.1.2 Analysis at the end of the data collection period

At the end of the data collection period, you need to come together as a team for a couple of days to discuss the findings. It is probably most useful if the whole team works together on this. Remember to look for not only similarities in the information, but also differences. Differences can help you understand how distinct population groups are affected by the shock in different ways and will help you plan a better intervention. The purpose of the analysis is to develop a finalised causal analysis for the assessment. The objectives of the analysis are to determine:

- which causes of malnutrition have arisen as a result of the emergency and are therefore acute in nature (rather than long-term, chronic causes of malnutrition)?
- what is the extent of nutritional risk posed by the cause? Will the main causes of malnutrition continue to be a problem in the foreseeable future? Is an immediate response required to prevent excess mortality and malnutrition?

If you have collected some information using a questionnaire you will need to analyse this on the computer. Sections B3.10 and B3.11 describe how to present information on vaccination coverage and morbidity collected by the questionnaire method.

The output you should aim for is a description of the causes of malnutrition in the emergency.[1] It may be helpful to present this information in the form of the conceptual framework so that the logic flowing between the causes – from basic causes to the outcome of malnutrition and mortality – can easily be seen. The most important causes (those which are acute and pose high nutritional risk) should be highlighted in a different colour. The sources for the information on the causal framework should also be highlighted. Any inconsistencies in the information which could not be resolved during the data collection should be clear on the framework. You should finalise your seasonal calendar by including events which will follow the assessment.

A5.2 Deciding which causes are important

Deciding which factor is an important cause of malnutrition can be difficult. This is because there are not always agreed standards for what is a normal or acceptable level of a problem. The important causes in an emergency nutrition assessment are those which result directly from the emergency and those which pose high nutritional risk. The following sections provide some guidance and provide internationally recognised benchmarks to help you decide which causes are the most important.

---

[1] The flipchart which you developed for the causes before the emergency identifies the long-term causes and is useful for developing recommendations.

A5.2.1 Information on immediate causes

Health status

Confirmation of an outbreak is not always straightforward because clear definitions of outbreak thresholds do not exist for all diseases:

- diseases for which one case may indicate an outbreak include cholera, measles, yellow fever, shigella, viral haemorrhagic fevers
- less specific definitions exist for malaria, although an increase in the number of cases above what is expected for the time of year among a defined population in a defined area may indicate an outbreak.

Remember that even a single case of measles is cause for concern and you should consider implementing a mass measles vaccination campaign immediately.

Other than for outbreaks, morbidity data can be difficult to interpret because there are often no 'norms' with which to compare the information you have collected.[2] To illustrate this point, imagine you have asked the mothers of all children about whether or not their child had diarrhoea in the past two weeks and 20% of the mothers replied that their children did indeed have diarrhoea. How do we know how to interpret this? Was does this figure of 20% mean? Unless you have information (normally from the MoH) on what the 'norm' for the prevalence of diarrhoea is in that particular season, the 20% figure is meaningless because you don't know if it is typical or not. The interpretation of morbidity data is further complicated by the fact that the prevalence of diarrhoea will depend on access to health care. It is because of these difficulties in interpreting morbidity data from questionnaires that this manual recommends obtaining information on morbidity from the MoH (subsection A4.5.2) rather than through questionnaires.

Contrary to the problems described above, morbidity information from interviews with the MoH or mothers' groups can be useful in helping you to think about the causes of malnutrition. If, for example, the MoH staff and mothers' groups all reported that there had been a substantial increase in the amount of diarrhoea in the area among young children in the weeks prior to the survey because some important sources of water had dried up, you could conclude that this was an important contribution to the development of malnutrition and you could make recommendations to improve the situation.

---

[2] Information on national norms is often available from a recent demographic health survey or the MoH.

Food intake

If, in your analysis of secondary or primary data sources, you find that part of the population is facing a food deficit, then you can assume the population's food intake (in terms of either energy or micronutrients) is a problem.

A5.2.2 Information on food security

As for food intake, if in your analysis of secondary or primary data sources, you find that part of the population is facing a food deficit, then you can assume the population's food security is a problem.

To a certain extent, you must use your own judgement to determine how important food security is in the causal framework. Two important things to consider are: (i) the extent of the deficit; and, (ii) the types of coping mechanisms employed by the population.

If the food deficit is very large then it is likely that shortage of food is playing an important part in the development of malnutrition. For example, displaced populations that have had to leave all their food stocks behind are likely to be in dire need of food. Remember that food shortages are common for some populations in the developing world at certain times of year. If you undertake your assessment prior to the harvest and the population has a small deficit of food it may not pose a high nutritional risk warranting an urgent response.

As described in Chapter A1, people adopt a range of strategies (coping mechanisms) to deal with reductions in food availability and access. As the process continues towards the later stages of food insecurity, coping mechanisms become exhausted and the priorities of the individual and community shift towards survival. Information on coping strategies can be extremely helpful in deciding the level of nutritional risk posed by the emergency. If a large section of the population is practising unusual coping mechanisms, particularly strategies that will affect their long-term ability to survive, then this is an indication that the situation is severe.

A5.2.3 Information on public health

The WHO recommends that measles vaccination rate should be at least 90% to prevent an epidemic. If the vaccination coverage is estimated to be less than 90% a mass measles vaccination campaign for children six months to 15 years (including administration of vitamin A to children aged 6–59 months) is recommended. A measles outbreak poses a real risk to the population's nutritional status. Vitamin A deficiency is associated with increased mortality, especially when children have low weight for height. WHO/Unicef recommend that children living in the developing world, in food insecure conditions, should receive a vitamin A supplement twice a year. If the data indicates that the population has not received vitamin A in the past six months then you should consider implementing a vitamin A supplementation campaign.

BCG vaccinations are usually given during routine work on an expanded programme of immunisation (EPI), and hence the rate may give an indication of how well the primary health care system is working – if the rate is very low then you can assume that EPI is not strong. Not every individual who has been vaccinated with BCG develops a scar and there is some evidence that if children are vaccinated in infancy a significant proportion do not have a permanent scar. It is likely that BCG scar therefore underestimates vaccination coverage but it is widely accepted as a useful measure nonetheless. Attendance at health facilities can help determine the utilisation rate. There is no definitive threshold for utilisation, as this will vary from context to context, and often from season to season. However, it usually increases significantly among displaced populations. Among stable populations, utilisation rates are approximately 0.5–1.0 new consultations/person/year. Among displaced populations, an average of 4.0 new consultations/person/year may be expected. A rate which is lower than expected may indicate inadequate access to health facilities (because of insecurity, distance, cost or poor capacity of health services). A rate which is higher may suggest over-utilisation due to a specific public health problem (eg, an epidemic), or under-estimation of the size of the target population.

Ideally, all people should have safe and equitable access to a sufficient quantity of water for drinking, cooking, and personal and domestic hygiene. Public water points should be sufficiently close to households to enable the use of the minimum water requirement. People should have adequate numbers of latrines, sufficiently close to their dwellings, to allow them rapid, safe and acceptable access at all times of the day and night. Latrines should be sited, designed, constructed and maintained in such a way as to be comfortable, hygienic and safe to use. More specific guidelines are given by The Sphere Project (2004):

- Average water use for drinking, cooking and personal hygiene in any household should be at least 15 litres per person per day.
- The maximum distance from any household to the nearest water point should be 500 metres.
- Queuing time at a water source should be no more than 15 minutes.
- It should take no more than three minutes to fill a 20-litre container.
- Water sources and systems should be maintained such that appropriate quantities of water are available consistently or on a regular basis.
- A maximum of 20 people should use each latrine and latrines should be no more than 50 metres from dwellings.
- Latrines should be used in the most hygienic way and children's faeces should be disposed of immediately and hygienically.

- Pit latrines and soakaways (for most soils) should be at least 30 metres from any groundwater source and the bottom of any latrine should be at least 1.5 metres above the water table. Drainage or spillage from defecation systems must not run towards any surface water source or shallow groundwater source.

Inadequate access to clean water poses a major nutritional risk in all settings. When people are displaced or living in overcrowded conditions, poor sanitation also poses a major risk.

A5.2.4 Information on the social and care environment

In general, there are no standards, or norms, for caring practices because they are so culture and context specific. This makes it difficult to interpret the information you collect on caring practices.

Example A5.2

Bottle feeding and the use of breastmilk substitutes in an emergency, particularly during displacement, pose a major nutritional risk. For example, during the 1991 refugee crisis in Northern Iraq, the crude mortality rate among Kurdish refugees was reported to be 3/10,000/day. Two-thirds of the deaths occurred among children aged five years or younger, and half among infants younger than one year. Most deaths were due to diarrhoea, dehydration and resulting malnutrition. Infant feeding practices, particularly use of infant formula, combined with poor, inadequate water and sanitation, were implicated in the high incidence of diarrhoeal disease. While infant formula can be particularly dangerous, sub-optimal infant feeding practices, such as low rates of exclusive breastfeeding, are widespread in non-emergency contexts and are therefore unlikely to represent a new cause of malnutrition in emergency. Nevertheless, interventions to improve rates of exclusive breastfeeding in emergencies may reduce nutritional and mortality risk considerably for young children. Sudden changes in access to foods typically given to young children can be an important cause of malnutrition – in pastoralist populations, for example, reduced access to cow's or goat's milk can present high nutritional risk.

Acute problems in the social and care environment that might create a high risk of malnutrition may result from declines in food security. For example, a prolonged drought resulting in a severe shortage of firewood for cooking could cause some households to stop cooking every day. They are only able to cook food once every two days. The food is then stored in unhygienic conditions. This has resulted in the food going bad and people becoming ill. The lack of access to fuel in this situation may be an important cause of malnutrition.

Interpreting information on the dependency ratio (or effective dependency ratio) can help provide information on the capacity of households to look after themselves. Extremely high dependency ratios may be an important cause of malnutrition due to their knock-on effects on food security and the capacity to provide nutritional care for children and women. The following classification can be used to interpret dependency ratios, although there are no internationally agreed cut-offs for determining dependency ratios:

Category	Ratio	Dependants per active adult
Low	0–0.33	Less than one dependant per active adult
Moderate	0.34–0.66	One or two dependants per active adult
High	0.67–0.99	Three or more dependants per active adult
Extremely high	1	No active adults

(source: SADC, 2003)

An analysis of subgroups of the population who are at heightened risk of malnutrition may identify some groups in urgent need of assistance. Separated children and people excluded from receiving assistance are two groups which may face acute nutritional risk.

A5.2.5 Basic causes

Displacement, repeated and prolonged shocks are likely to pose the greatest nutritional risk (see Section A1.4).

Summary

- Analysis of the primary data collected on the causes of malnutrition should take place during the assessment and be discussed among the team in order to revise the pre-assessment causal framework and seasonal calendar. Data gathered through quantitative methods should be analysed on the computer.
- The final analysis of the causes of malnutrition should seek to identify the most important causes of malnutrition: that is, those that are acute and result from the emergency, and those that present the greatest nutritional risk and may require urgent intervention to address.

Part B
Assessing the prevalence of malnutrition

In this section of the manual we look at how to estimate the prevalence of malnutrition using an anthropometric survey. Chapter B1 provides an explanation of how to measure malnutrition in an emergency-affected population and looks at topics such as which age group to measure, which measurements to take, etc. This chapter should be read in conjunction with Appendix S2 which provides practical tips on how to take the measurements. Chapter B2 describes the different types of sampling methods commonly employed for anthropometric surveys. Finally, Chapter B3 explains how to produce and present results from the anthropometric data.

So, at the end of Part B you should have understood how to produce estimates of the prevalence of malnutrition. This data is then used, in conjunction with estimates of mortality and information about the causes of the malnutrition, to make recommendations about how to improve the nutritional situation of the emergency-affected population – covered in Part D.

Chapter B1
Anthropometric measurements and indices

As stated in Chapter A1, malnutrition is caused by a lack of nutrients resulting from ill-health or inadequate food intake. Assessments of malnutrition using functional and metabolic tests are neither practical nor efficient in an emergency situation. Instead, anthropometric measurements (measurements of body proportions such as weight and height) are used to give an approximation of the nutrition status of a population, or to monitor the growth and development of an individual.

At an individual level, anthropometric data is used to determine whether or not a person is malnourished. In turn, this information may be used to decide whether or not the individual should be included in a supplementary feeding programme or treated for severe malnutrition. The information is also used to decide when to discharge the individual from a feeding programme.

At the population level, anthropometric data is used either in a survey to assess what proportion of a population is malnourished, or as a surveillance tool to follow the nutritional situation of a population over time. This type of information helps planners to decide whether or not an intervention is required at the population level.

This chapter describes the anthropometric measurements and indices that should be used in a population survey.

B1.1 Which age group?

In emergencies, weight loss among children aged 6–59 months is usually taken as a proxy indicator for the general health and well-being of the entire community. This assumes that children aged 6–59 months are more vulnerable than other age groups to external factors (such as food shortages and illness) and the nutrition status of these children is more sensitive to change than that of adults in many populations. Also, in practice this group is much easier to measure than other population groups. This means that surveys of children aged 6–59 months are trying to draw conclusions about the situation of the whole population, not just young children. Therefore, for nutrition assessments in emergencies, it is usual to measure only children aged 6–59 months.[1]

---

[1] In some places the exact age of children might not be known. In this situation, you are advised to develop a local calendar to estimate age. Failing this you may use a height cut-off which approximates to the upper age limit. This is discussed in detail in subsections S1.2.1, Annex S1.

The anthropometric indicators used to assess acute malnutrition in adolescents, adults and older people have not yet been internationally agreed and so the measurement of malnutrition in these age groups is more problematic. Sections B1.7 and B1.8 consider when it might be appropriate to measure other age groups (less than six months and over five years).

B1.2 Measuring malnutrition in children aged 6–59 months: nutrition indices and indicators

B1.2.1 Nutrition indices and indicators

Nutrition indices are a combination of measurements compared with a reference. In order to determine the nutrition status of an individual, his or her weight, height and age must be recorded. The presence of bilateral oedema should also be noted. Appendix S2 describes how to measure height, weight, mid-upper arm circumference and oedema in children aged 6–59 months. Specifications for measuring equipment are also given. Appendix S3 describes how to train workers to obtain standardised measurements.

Information on a child's weight, height, or age alone does not give sufficient information to determine whether or not the child is malnourished. For example, knowing that a child weighs 10kg is useful only if the height or age is given as well. Furthermore, the combination of weight and height make sense only when compared with a normal value, derived from a reference population.

When body measurements are compared with a reference value they are called nutrition indices. Three commonly used nutrition indices are weight-for-height (WFH), height-for-age (HFA) and weight-for-age (WFA). The mid-upper arm circumference (MUAC) is also used in assessing malnutrition in emergencies (see Section B1.4).

Weight-for-height	reflects recent weight loss or gain. It is the best indicator of wasting and so is the indicator used for determining **acute malnutrition.**
Height-for-age	reflects skeletal growth, and is the best indicator of stunting. This is the indicator used for determining **chronic malnutrition.**
Weight-for-age	is a composite index, which reflects either wasting or stunting, or a combination of both. Rapidly changing WFA can be assumed to be the result of changing WFH, while low WFA among older children is more likely to be the result of low HFA. Hence, this is the indicator used for determining if a child is **underweight.**

| MUAC | reflects recent weight loss or gain. It is used as an indicator of wasting and **acute malnutrition**.
source: Young and Jaspars, 1995 |

Nutrition indicators are an interpretation of nutrition indices based on cut-off points. Whereas indices are simply a figure, indicators represent an interpretation of the indices. Nutrition indicators are used for making a judgement or assessment.

A nutrition indicator is a tool to measure the clinical phenomena of malnutrition. A good indicator is one that detects, as much as possible, those at risk of death (sensitivity) without including too many of those not at risk (specificity). A good indicator of malnutrition should also be functionally meaningful, in other words, a useful indicator will be related to the risk of morbidity.

B1.2.2 The reference population curves

In order to assess malnutrition as defined by WFH, HFA and WFA, individual measurements are compared with an international reference value for a normal US child population (NCHS/WHO/CDC reference table, WHO, 1983). These reference values were calculated from data collected by the National Centre for Health Statistics (NCHS) in the United States in 1975. The World Health Organization (WHO) adopted the NCHS references in 1980.[2]

An international reference is needed to allow comparison of nutrition status of populations in different parts of the world. There is evidence that growth patterns in well-fed children in a favourable environment are reasonably similar in all ethnic groups, at least up to five years of age. The variation between ethnic groups is relatively minor compared with the large worldwide variation that relates to health, nutrition and socio-economic status.

Some countries have considered developing their own growth reference curves. However, this is a very costly and time-consuming process. In addition, in developing countries the reference curves will need to be updated regularly to take into account secular trends (increases in height between generations due to improved nutrition). The WHO, therefore, recommends that one single international reference be observed.[3]

---

[2] The NCHS reference has certain disadvantages. These include the fact that the references were drawn from measurements made only on US children (no other nationalities were included) and that most of these children were bottle-fed infants. It is now recognised that growth patterns are different in breast-fed and bottle-fed children.

[3] The WHO is in the process of developing new reference curves from a multi-country study involving only breast-fed children from different ethnic groups.

The NCHS reference population should not be considered as reflecting an 'ideal' nutrition status, given its limitations (see footnote) but should be used as a tool to compare the nutrition status from different regions, or the nutrition status of one population over time.

The NCHS references for children aged 0–59 months can be found in Appendix S4.

B1.3 Expression of nutrition indices and indicators

Before reading this section make sure you are familiar with the basic statistics described in Appendix S5. Anthropometric indices or indicators can be expressed in terms of percentage of the median or z-scores.[4]

B1.3.1 The percentage of the median and reference population

The index of weight-for-height median (WHM) compares the weight of the measured child with the median weight of children of the same height in the reference population. The calculation of a WHM for each child is based on:
a)   the child's weight
b)   the median weight for children of the same height and sex in the reference population

$$WHM = \frac{individual's\ weight}{median\ reference\ weight} \times 100$$

Example B1.1
In a nutritional survey, a male child of 92cm weighs 12.1kg. In Table S4.1 (Appendix S4), it can be seen that the median weight for a boy of height 92cm is 13.7kg.

$$WHM = \frac{12.1}{13.7} \times 100$$

$$= 88.3\%$$

---

[4] Percentiles are also used. The percentile is the rank position of an individual on a given reference table. Because percentiles are used primarily for the 'road to health' chart in growth monitoring and are not usually used in emergency assessments, we will not be discussing them here.

B1.3.2 The z-score and reference population

A z-score is a measure of how far a child is from the median weight of the reference distribution for children of the same height, taking into consideration the standard deviation of the reference distribution. More technically, it is the deviation of an individual value from the median of the reference distribution. The calculation of a weight-for-height z-score (WHZ) for each child is based on:

a) the child's weight
b) the median weight for children of the same height and sex in the reference population
c) the standard deviation for the distribution of weights in the reference population for children of the same height and sex (because the standard deviation of a distribution increases as children get older, you need to use the standard deviation for the reference distribution of children of the same height).

$$\text{WHZ} = \frac{\text{individual's weight} - \text{median reference weight}}{\text{standard deviation of weight for the reference population}}$$

Example B1.2
In a nutrition survey, a male child of 84cm weighs 9.9kg. Referring to Table S4.1 (Appendix S4), the reference median weight for boys of height 84cm is 11.7kg. From Table S4.2 (Appendix S4) we can also see that the standard deviation for the reference distribution for boys of height 84cm is 0.908. Using these values you can calculate a z-score for this child in the sample.

$$\text{WHZ} = \frac{9.9 - 11.7}{0.908}$$

$$= -1.98$$

B1.3.3 Mean weight-for-height percentage (of the median)

The mean weight-for-height percentage of the median (WHM) is sometimes used as a way to describe the nutrition status of a population. The mean WHM is the statistical mean of the individual WHM values in a group. This indicates the overall nutritional status in the group.

$$\text{mean WHM} = \frac{\text{sum of WHM values in the group}}{\text{total number of children in the group}}$$

This indicator provides a summary of the nutrition status values of all children in a group. It provides an average figure and may be useful to compare the nutrition status of groups of children over time or between different groups of children. The prevalence of low WHM and WHZ should always be reported in an emergency nutrition assessment; mean WHM can be optionally reported.

B1.3.4 Mean weight-for-height z-score

The mean weight-for-height z-score (WHZ) is sometimes used as a way to describe the nutrition status of a population. The mean WHZ is the statistical mean of the individual WHZ values in a group. This indicates the overall nutritional status in the group.

$$\text{mean WHZ} = \frac{\text{sum of WHZ values in the group}}{\text{total number of children in the group}}$$

This indicator provides a summary of the nutrition status values of all children in a group. It provides an average figure and may be useful to compare the nutrition status of groups of children over time or between different groups of children. Percentage of the median and z-scores should always be reported in an emergency nutrition assessment; like the mean WHM, the mean WHZ can be optionally reported.

B1.4 Definitions of acute malnutrition in children aged 6–59 months

Weight-for-height
The WFH nutrition index is appropriate in emergency assessments because it reflects short-term growth failure or acute malnutrition related to weight loss (wasting). Thus, WFH is the most commonly used nutrition index in emergency nutrition surveys. This is because it can tell us about the current situation of the population. A further advantage of WFH is that it does not involve age. Age is often difficult to determine, especially in emergency situations and can be unreliable. WFH is also used as a criterion for admission into and discharge from feeding programmes and to monitor the evolution of the nutrition status of a child enrolled in a feeding programme.

Oedema
The presence of oedema should also be assessed during emergency assessments. Oedema is caused by the retention of water and sodium in the extracellular spaces. Bilateral pitting oedema (oedema on both feet) is the key indicator of

kwashiorkor. Hence, the presence of oedema on both feet indicates severe malnutrition. All children with bilateral oedema are regarded as being severely acutely malnourished, irrespective of their WFH. Oedema should, therefore, always be used as a criterion for admission into therapeutic feeding programmes. The diagnosis of oedema is described in Section S2.2.5, Appendix S2.

MUAC

Mid-upper arm circumference (MUAC) measures the muscle mass of the upper arm. It is a rapid and effective predictor of risk of death when below 110mm in children aged 12–59 months. However, there are drawbacks to using MUAC in emergencies. The chance of inaccurate measurement is high due to differing techniques, and clear and agreed reference values to interpret the results do not yet exist (see subsection B1.4.4).

Moderate, severe and global malnutrition

Acute malnutrition is classified at individual level as normal, moderate acute and severe acute malnutrition. At population level, the prevalence of malnutrition is expressed as severe acute malnutrition and global acute malnutrition. Global acute malnutrition expresses the sum of severe acute malnutrition and moderate acute malnutrition.

| Prevalence of global acute malnutrition | = | Prevalence of moderate acute malnutrition | + | Prevalence of severe acute malnutrition |

Various different cut-off points, which employ different nutritional indices, are used to define acute malnutrition in children aged 6–59 months. The most commonly used cut-offs are defined below.

B1.4.1 Weight-for-height cut-offs

The cut-offs in table B1.1 are used to define acute malnutrition according to weight-for-height measurements:

- This means that any child with a WHM less than 80 per cent or a WHZ less than −2 is defined as acutely malnourished.
- Children with a WHM less than 80 per cent and more than or equal to 70 per cent, or a WHZ less than −2 and more than or equal to −3 are defined as moderately acutely malnourished.
- Children with a WHM of below 70 per cent or a WHZ of below −3 are defined as severely acutely malnourished.
- All children with bilateral oedema are severely acutely malnourished regardless of their WHM or WHZ.

Table B1.1 Definitions of acute malnutrition using weight-for-height and/or oedema in children aged 6–59 months

Acute malnutrition using WFH	Percentage of the median	Z-scores	Oedema
Severe	< 70 %	<– 3 z-scores	Yes/no
	>70 %	>– 3 z-scores	Yes
Moderate	< 80% to >= 70%	<– 2 z-scores to >= – 3 z-scores	No
Global	< 80%	<– 2 z-scores	Yes/no

These cut-offs can be used to diagnose whether or not an individual child is malnourished (and therefore should be admitted into a feeding programme), as well as to estimate the prevalence of malnutrition in a survey.

Example B1.3
The child described above in Example B1.1 who had a WHM of 88.3% is not acutely malnourished because his WHM falls above the cut-off point for acute malnutrition. Likewise, the child described in Example B1.2 is not acutely malnourished because his z-score is −1.98, which is above the cut-off. However, a child who had oedema or had a WHM <70% would be defined as severely acutely malnourished.

The cut-offs can also be used to estimate the prevalence of acute malnutrition in surveys using WHM and WHZ.

Example B1.4
A group of 905 children was measured in a survey. There was no oedema. Fifteen children had WHZ<−3 z-scores and 45 had WHZ<−2 z-scores and >=− 3 z-scores.

$$\text{prevalence of severe acute malnutrition} = \frac{\text{number of severely malnourished children}}{\text{total number of children}} \times 100$$

$$= \frac{15}{905} \times 100$$

$$= 1.7\%$$

prevalence of moderate = number of moderately malnourished × 100
acute malnutrition   children
_____

total number of children

$$= \frac{45}{905} \times 100$$

$$= 5.0\%$$

prevalence of global acute = prevalence of severe acute malnutrition +
malnutrition   prevalence of moderate acute malnutrition

$$= 1.7 + 5.0$$

$$= 6.7\%.$$

B1.4.2 Percentage of the median or z-scores?

Different children are categorised as malnourished depending on whether percentage of the median or z-score is used to define malnutrition. If z-scores are used to define malnutrition then a greater number of taller (older) children will be defined as malnourished than if percentage of the median is used. Generally, if z-scores are used, the number of children classified as malnourished is higher than if the percentage of the median is used (see subsection D1.1.7 and figure B1.1).

Why is there a difference between z-scores and percentage of the median?

The standard deviation of weight is different for different heights in the reference population. At a low height the standard deviation of weight is quite small, at greater heights the standard deviation of weight is greater. This means that children of different heights have different standard deviations of weight in the reference population.

When you calculate the z-score you take into account three factors – the median measurement, the actual measurement, and the standard deviation for the specific measurement. So, the z-score takes into account the variation in the standard deviation. When you calculate the percentage of the median you only take into account two factors – the median measurement and the actual measurement. The percentage median does not take into account the variation in the standard deviation.

What this means is that the z-score is more statistically valid than the

Figure B1.1 <80% WFH compared to <–2 z-scores WFH of the NCHS reference population

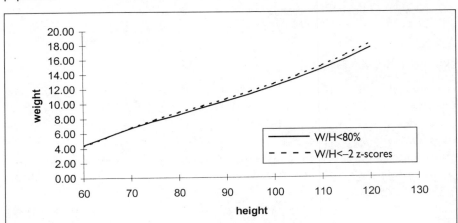

percentage of the median. Using z-scores, a taller (older) child is as likely to be classified as malnourished as a shorter (younger) child. This is not true for percentage of the median. Thus, the WHO recommends the use of z-scores to measure children (WHO, 2000).

The concept of the percentage of the median is easier to explain than that of z-scores because it does not require knowledge of standard deviations. Percentage of the median is also easier to calculate. A further advantage of percentage of the median is that several recent studies have shown that it is a better predictor of mortality than z-score.

Percentage of the median therefore has more practical operational advantages, whereas the advantages of z-scores lies in their statistical precision (see also subsection D1.1.1).

When to use z-scores or percentage of the median

- Anthropometric survey results should be given in both z-scores and percentage of the median.
- Admission criteria for entrance to a feeding centre are usually defined using percentage of the median (because of mortality risk and ease of calculation).
- When you are making decisions about whether or not to intervene at a given prevalence of malnutrition, you should look at the prevalence of both severe and global acute malnutrition measured in terms of z-scores and/or oedema, in conjunction with the mortality rate and the causes of malnutrition. This is discussed further in Chapter D1.

B1.4.3 Mean weight-for-height cut-offs

The mean WHM or WHZ cannot be used to define malnutrition in individuals. There are no internationally accepted cut-offs for mean WHM or WHZ.

B1.4.4 MUAC cut-offs

As stated above, MUAC cut-offs have not yet been internationally agreed. Some years ago, the MUACs of children (both boys and girls) between the ages of one and five years were assumed to remain roughly constant, ie, MUAC was thought to be independent of age in this group. This assumption was based on measurements from a small sample of Polish children. This meant that the same fixed cut-offs to denote malnutrition was used for a girl aged 12 months and a boy aged 59 months.

More recent research has shown that MUAC varies by age and sex among children aged 1–5 years and during this period MUAC increases normally by up to 2cm. This means that well-nourished children aged four years have higher MUACs than well-nourished children aged one year. There are also considerable sex differences in MUAC among children aged <24 months.

For these reasons, the WHO now recommends the use of reference data for MUAC according to age, sex and height. These are compiled in tables with median and z-score values[5] and based on the NCHS reference data. MUAC for height is the preferred MUAC indicator for use in populations where age is difficult to determine.[6]

Using MUAC in emergency programmes

MUAC has three current functions in emergency programmes:

1. to determine the prevalence of malnutrition as a rapid alternative to WFH
2. to act as a first-stage screening process for selective feeding programmes – eg, supplementary feeding or therapeutic feeding centres (TFCs)
3. to admit children to TFCs.

---

[5] See *The Management of Nutrition in Major Emergencies*, WHO 2000.
[6] MUAC for height can be simply measured using the QUAC stick. QUAC sticks have been used for some time but have in the past used a range of reference data sets other than the NCHS. QUAC sticks can be easily constructed (see *The Management of Nutrition in Major Emergencies*, WHO 2000.

Using MUAC to determine the prevalence of malnutrition as an alternative to WFH

Different agencies recommend different cut-offs of MUAC to determine moderate/severe acute malnutrition (see table B1.2).

Table B1.2 MUAC cut-offs recommended by different agencies

Agency	Age group	Moderate acute malnutrition	Severe acute malnutrition
The Sphere Project (2004)[7]	6–59 mths	110–125mm	<110mm
Médecins Sans Frontières (MSF, in press)	12–59 mths		<110mm
	<12 mths		<100mm, or <110mm in poor clinical condition
WHO (2000)	6–59 mths	Differs according to age	Differs according to age

The use of a single MUAC cut-off point to classify children aged 12–59 months as malnourished will not result in the same children being classified as malnourished using WFH methods. This is because:

- MUAC is dependent on both age and height and will therefore identify more young children and fewer older children as malnourished compared with the WFH method. The sensitivity and specificity of MUAC with a fixed cut-off varies according to the age of the child. Using MUAC for height reduces the sensitivity of MUAC for younger children and increases the sensitivity for older children[8]
- the ability of MUAC to correctly identify the same children as WFH as malnourished also depends on the underlying prevalence of malnutrition. The sensitivity of lower MUAC cut-offs will increase in populations with a higher prevalence of malnutrition.

Use of MUAC for screening

At the start of a feeding programme MUAC can be used to screen for malnutrition when large numbers of children are involved. Children with a MUAC less than a

---

[7] MUAC is recommended for use by The Sphere Project as part of two-stage screening rather than alone in surveys.

[8] *sensitivity*: the ability of MUAC to identify true cases of malnutrition as identified by WFH
specificity: the ability of MUAC to identify true negative cases of malnutrition as identified by WFH.

given cut-off are then referred for height and weight measurements. The purpose of this screening is to speed up the process of admission (weight and height measurements take longer to complete) into selective feeding programmes.

However, where there are low levels of malnutrition a relatively high MUAC cut-off (such as 14cm) may be needed to ensure that the screening identifies most malnourished children. In this situation it may be quicker to take a single WFH measure rather than do two-stage screening. If you intend to use MUAC as part of two-stage screening, you should determine the appropriate MUAC cut-offs which should be used for different age groups. The following steps should be followed.

1. A sample of 150–200 children should be taken. This does not have to be a random or a representative sample, but it is important that it includes children of different ages, sexes and nutritional status. The easiest way may be to go house-to-house in a single village.
2. The sex, age, height, weight and MUAC should be recorded for each child.
3. The programme screen.exe should be installed from the CD-ROM which comes with this manual. After installation, start the programme. Open the menu entitled 'Screen'. Highlight and click on 'new file' and give a name to the dataset which you are about to enter. Then go back to the 'screen menu' and highlight and click on 'Enter data'. Press enter and select the name of your dataset. Then enter the variables (age, sex, MUAC, weight and height). When you have finished press F10. Return to the same 'screen menu' and highlight and click on 'report'. Then select your dataset and allow the computer to make the necessary calculations. It is advisable to create separate files for children <12 months and children >12 months, since the MUACs differ considerably between these two age groups. This will mean that ultimately you have two separate MUAC cut-offs in use for the screening of these two different age groups.
4. You can interpret the results in the following way. The left-hand column indicates possible MUAC cut-offs which you could use in two-stage screening (to identify children who may be malnourished <80% WHM). In the second column is the sensitivity associated with each MUAC value. For example, if the sensitivity for a MUAC cut-off of 137mm is 0.70 it means that 70% of your children <80% WHM will be identified with this cut-off but 30% will be missed using this cut-off. The third column shows the specificity. If the specificity for a MUAC cut-off of 137cm is 0.69 it means that 69% of the children which you refer for WFH measurement will actually not meet the WHM criteria for entry into programmes (ie, they will be 80% WHM or more). It is recommended that you aim to have a high level of sensitivity (>0.8) so that you do not miss eligible children, but you need to be aware that this involves measuring both MUAC and WFH for some children who

will ultimately not be eligible. This is why it is really only saves time to do MUAC screening first if you have very large numbers of children or you are screening in the community first for referral to a centre (where you do not have scales and height boards).

5.   Press F10 to quit.

Admission of children into a TFC

Research has shown that children's MUAC is closely correlated with mortality in some circumstances. Indeed, several studies have shown that MUAC is a better indicator of mortality in either a community or a hospital for severely malnourished children, than WFH. In addition, MUAC is not affected by oedema or heavy parasite loads. This is why it may be important to allow children with very low MUACs but higher WFH (because of parasite loads) into a feeding programme. Some international non-governmental organisations (NGOs) have, therefore, recommended that MUAC cut-offs be used as an additional entrance criterion to emergency nutrition programmes. There are two problems with this approach:

- There is no internationally agreed cut-off for MUACs (see table above).
- Recovery from malnutrition is usually measured by weight gain. This makes it difficult to decide when to discharge a child who is normally nourished according to WFH but not for MUAC.

Recommendations on the use of MUAC or WFH

- Do not use MUAC as an alternative to WFH in a nutritional survey. Because of the problems which have been associated with MUAC, it is not an indicator which is widely accepted as accurate by donors. Furthermore, since entry criteria for targeted feeding programmes are based on WFH, an MUAC cut-off which identified the same proportion of children as malnourished as WFH would need to be identified in advance for the specific population being measured.
- MUAC can be used in two-stage screening, although the cut-off needs to be investigated so that it has the highest levels of sensitivity for all age groups (using screen.exe). Two-stage screening using MUAC is only likely to present a cost saving (in staff time) in populations where acute malnutrition levels are high – eg, >15–20% – or where there are very large numbers of children.
- MUAC may be usefully gathered alongside WFH in a survey. This may provide additional information about the mortality risk in the population. But remember to always test measurement error for MUAC (see Appendix S3).
- Children with an MUAC <11cm should be admitted into therapeutic feeding

programmes (TFPs), as they can have a high risk of mortality or a big parasite load. Exit criteria for these children should follow the standard TFP protocols.

B1.4.5 Classification of nutrition status among acutely malnourished individuals

Several different classifications of nutrition status have been suggested in the past. Currently, the most widely used classification of nutrition status is based on WFH indices and oedema. Individuals with low WFH are defined as marasmic. Individuals who have oedema have kwashiorkor. Individuals who are both low WFH and have oedema suffer from marasmic kwashiorkor. Table B1.3 shows this classification.

Table B1.3 The Waterlow classification of acute malnutrition based on WFH and oedema

	<–2 z-score or <80% median	>= –2 z-score or >= 80% median
Oedema present	Marasmic kwashiorkor	Kwashiorkor
Oedema absent	Marasmic	Normal

This classification is important in emergency nutritional assessments because individuals with marasmic kwashiorkor have a higher risk of mortality than other groups. When planning an intervention, it is important to know what proportion of the population will need life-saving treatment. All emergency nutrition assessments should, therefore, present data based on this classification (see Chapter B3 for more details on this).

B1.5 Definition of chronic malnutrition in children aged 6–59 months

A child exposed to inadequate nutrition or bouts of disease for a long period of time will grow slowly. His or her height will be reduced, compared with other children of the same age who are not exposed to poor nutrition or disease, and so s/he will have low height-for-age (HFA). This is called stunting. Unlike wasting, the development of stunting is a slow, cumulative process. It may not be evident for some years, by which time nutrition may have improved (although, by two years of age, height deficits may be irreversible).

Stunting, or low HFA, is a measure of chronic malnutrition (longer-term malnutrition) and is therefore not always useful for describing the current situation. The long timescale over which HFA is affected makes it more useful for long-term planning and policy development than for emergencies. For example, it is useful for evaluating the effects of socio-economic change or development programmes in a certain place.

Apart from the fact that stunting represents chronic malnutrition, the very high levels of stunting in much of the developing world also mean that it is not useful in emergency assessments, or as a screening tool for entrance into emergency feeding programmes.

For the reasons described above, emergency assessments usually do not assess chronic malnutrition. Before attempting to collect data on chronic malnutrition in an emergency assessment you need to think carefully about how useful it will be.[9] Are you actually interested in the long-term, chronic deprivation of the area, or do you want to know only about the recent past? Also remember that HFA is only useful when exact ages are known (to the closest month). Incorrect age data will make the HFA data meaningless. In a population that does not know the ages of its children (as with many populations in the developing world), correct age data can be difficult to obtain and may take a long time to collect.

B1.6 Definition of underweight in children aged 6–59 months

Low WFA can be due to low WFH, or low HFA, or both. Therefore, WFA reflects both long-term malnutrition and recent malnutrition. Because of this mix, WFA is not useful for specifically assessing acute or chronic malnutrition. WFA is used for growth monitoring of individual children using the 'road to health' chart.[10] WFA should not be used either in emergency nutrition assessments or as a criterion for the selection of children for feeding programmes.

B1.7 When to measure the nutritional status of people aged more than five years

Emergency assessments focus on children aged 6–59 months because, in general, the nutrition status of the under-five population has been shown to be a good proxy for the nutrition status of the wider community. Surveys including other age groups are more complex and require greater technical expertise than surveys assessing only children aged 6–59 months.

It is not always appropriate to assess malnutrition among for older children, adolescents, adults or older people in emergency situations. However, there are

---

[9] The most commonly used HFA cut-offs are given in Section S1.4, Appendix S1 for information purposes.
[10] The most commonly used WFA cut-offs are given in Section S2.5, Appendix S2 for information purposes.

some situations when it may be appropriate to consider assessing the nutrition status of these age groups (ACC/SCN, 2001). This could be for example if:

- there is an increase in the crude mortality rate (CMR) compared with under-five mortality rates (suggesting that the over-five population is more vulnerable than the under-fives)
- age groups other than those under-five are worse affected by certain diseases, for example, in contexts of high HIV/AIDS prevalence
- there is reasonable doubt that the nutrition status of young children reflects the rest of the population's nutritional situation. For example, in populations where cultural traditions mean that young child feeding has precedence over that of the parents and other age groups, it may be reasonable to suspect that older adults are particularly vulnerable to malnutrition
- many adults or older children attempt to enrol in selective feeding programmes or present themselves at health facilities
- if credible anecdotal reports of adult or adolescent under-nutrition are received
- there is low coverage of food aid in dependent populations
- the data are required as an advocacy tool to lever resources to address the needs of specific at risk groups.

B1.7.1 Pre-requisites for surveying other age groups

Surveys of other age groups should not be undertaken unless certain pre-requisites have been met.

- A thorough contextual analysis of the situation must be undertaken. This should include an analysis of the causes of malnutrition (see Part A). Only if the results of this analysis indicate that the over-five (and/or young infant) population is vulnerable should a nutrition survey for this age group be considered.
- Technical expertise must be available to ensure quality of data collection, adequate analysis and correct interpretation of results.
- The resource and/or opportunity costs of including other age groups in a survey should be considered.
- Clear and well-documented objectives of the survey are formulated.

B1.7.2 Indicators used to measure malnutrition in other age groups

There are no internationally accepted definitions of acute malnutrition using anthropometry in people aged more than 59 months. This is partly because ethnic differences in growth start to become apparent after five years of age. That is, a healthy child from Bangladesh may not grow in exactly the same way as a healthy Sudanese child. This means it is difficult to use only one reference population to compare all ethnic groups. A further reason is that, in most circumstances, information on the nutrition status of the group aged 6–59 months is sufficient for planners to make their decisions and so, to date, there has been little research on defining malnutrition in other age groups.

In major nutritional emergencies, however, it may be necessary to include older children, adolescents or adults in nutrition assessments or nutrition programmes. Therefore, indicators of malnutrition for these age groups are sometimes necessary. Research on defining the most suitable indicators of malnutrition for people aged more than 59 months is currently being undertaken by several agencies.

Early research (and many of the current handbooks) favoured the body mass index (BMI) which is defined as weight/height^2 (kg/m^2) as the most useful measure of adult malnutrition. However, recent research has shown that the BMI is influenced by body shape (in particular the sitting height to standing height ratio), which varies by ethnic group and is also subject to considerable intra-population variation. This makes it difficult to define a universal BMI cut-off point below which we can state that an adult is malnourished. Currently, the most promising indicator of adult malnutrition is a combination of a MUAC cut-off in conjunction with clinical and social signs. However, this information may well change in the next few years as more research is undertaken.

Given all the problems associated with measuring people over 59 months Save the Children UK has decided that it is not appropriate to describe current techniques in these guidelines. Instead, up-to-date information on how to measure height, weight, MUAC and oedema in older children, adolescents, adults and older people can be obtained from Save the Children's head office.[11]

B1.8 Measurement of malnutrition in infants aged less than six months

Most of the current guidelines on nutrition assessment do not include the measurement of young infants (children aged <6 months). One of the main reasons for this exclusion has been the assumption that malnutrition will be rare among this age group as they are usually breastfed and hence will be protected from malnutrition. Traditionally, lactating mothers are admitted to selective

---

[11] Documents on how to measure adult and adolescent malnutrition can also be found at: www.unsystem.org/scn/archives/adults/index.htm, www.unsystem.org/scn/archives/adolescentss/ index.htm and on the CD-ROM attached to this manual.

feeding programmes and it is assumed that by improving the nutritional status of the mother you will also improve the nutritional status of the breastfeeding infant. However, in some situations malnutrition has been found to be a significant problem in this age group.

Where nutritional problems are suspected among this age group, it may be appropriate to establish the prevalence of malnutrition in the under-6 month population and assess the main factors leading to malnutrition in this age group. This is important because the mortality rates of malnourished young infants are generally very high.

B1.8.1 Difficulties in assessment of malnutrition in young infants

The assessment of nutritional status in children under-6 months is, however, difficult for the following reasons.

Taking the measurements

- It is difficult to straighten small infants in order to get accurate measurements of length with a standard measuring board.
- The scales normally used in nutrition surveys (the Salter scale) have 100g calibrations. This may lead to imprecision in weight measurements for this age group (10g calibrations would be more suitable).
- Some survey staff may be afraid to take measurements of small babies because they are not used to handling such small infants and worry about hurting them.

Use of NCHS references

- NCHS standards for this age are for bottle-fed babies, who grow more quickly in the early months than breastfed children so it is not appropriate to compare the growth of breastfed babies with the reference standards. However, the WHO is developing appropriate references, which will be available in 2004.
- The NCHS growth references start at 49cm of length but some children are born smaller than this.

Interpreting the findings

- WHZ is less sensitive than WHM for infants less than 65cm in length – ie, fewer malnourished children will be identified if z-scores are used. This can be a problem because very young infants have a high mortality risk. It is therefore appropriate to ensure that percentage of the median is used in the interpretation of the prevalence of malnutrition in this age group (see figure B1.1).

- It is difficult to identify diarrhoea in breastfed babies. Normal definitions of diarrhoea are not appropriate.
- Malnutrition in young infants is linked to intrauterine growth retardation and not just the post-natal environment.

B1.8.2 Recommendations about assessing young infant malnutrition

These are some general recommendations to consider when deciding whether or not to include young infants in nutrition programmes or assessments.

When to include infants in a nutrition assessment

If you suspect there is a problem of wasting in this group then young infants should be included in a nutrition assessment. Situations that might lead you to expect a problem include:

- if the rate of exclusive breastfeeding is low or breastfeeding practices have deteriorated as a consequence of the emergency
- if many infants are bottle-fed, especially in displaced populations
- when you receive reports of carers presenting young infants at selective feeding programmes for enrolment, or carers presenting this age group at health posts.

Assessments

If you decide to include infants in an emergency nutrition assessment, you should:

- measure length very carefully to the nearest 0.1cm
- measure weight to the nearest 10g (see Section S2.1, Appendix S2)
- check for oedema carefully (remember that a fat baby may look a little like a child with oedema)
- collect data on breastfeeding practices in this group if possible (see subsections A2.1.5 and A4.5.5).

You can then use the standard NCHS references (Section S4.1, Appendix S4) to assess whether or not the child is wasted. Even though the references are not ideal for this age group (see subsection B1.2.3) they are all that is available. Remember that oedema is also included in the definition of acute malnutrition in this age group.

If you are uncomfortable with taking length measurements in this age group then you can assess WFA only (see Section S2.5, Appendix S2 and Section S4.4, Appendix S4). But remember that the age in months needs to be very accurate.

Admission to therapeutic feeding programmes

If the results of the assessment indicate the need to admit children to a therapeutic feeding programme then you will need to consult relevant treatment protocols.

Summary

- Anthropometric measurements and indices are used to estimate the proportion of people who are malnourished in a given population. These indices are interpreted according to cut-offs representing different degrees of severity of malnutrition.
- Emergency nutrition assessments should focus on acute malnutrition as measured by weight-for-height and/or oedema, as this is the best reflection of short-term growth failure.
- All emergency nutrition assessments should report the prevalence of low weight-for-height and/or oedema as defined by the percentage of the median and z-scores. The reporting of mid-upper arm circumference data is optional.
- Children aged 6–59 months are best measured in emergency nutrition assessments because, in general, the nutritional status of this age group is a good proxy for the nutritional status of the wider community. In addition, measuring other age groups is much more difficult.
- Young infants should be included in an emergency nutrition assessment if there is a good reason to suspect that they have elevated rates of malnutrition because the associated mortality risk is very high.

Chapter B2
Sampling methodologies for anthropometric surveys

This chapter outlines the most common types of sampling methodologies appropriate for use in emergency nutrition assessments. It is extremely important that appropriate sampling methodologies are followed to ensure that results of nutrition assessments are comparable, both within a country and globally.

B2.1 Fundamentals of sampling

B2.1.1 Why take a sample?

If all the children aged 6–59 months from a given population were measured, we would get a precise picture of the nutritional status of the population. This is called a census, or exhaustive survey, and it is possible in a small population. However, an exhaustive survey is normally long, costly and difficult to carry out in a large population. Instead of surveying all the children, we normally survey only a subgroup of the population, called a sample, which 'represents' the whole population.

> **Example B2.1**
> An estimate of malnutrition is needed for a population of about 2,000–3,000 people. We can estimate that about 18–20% of the population are children below five years of age (400–600). In this case it is possible to measure all the eligible children. This is called an exhaustive survey.

> **Example B2.2**
> If we measured all children aged 6–59 months in a particular district we would know the exact prevalence of nutrition in the district. Imagine the total population of a district is estimated at 159,000 – this means there are about 31,800 children under five. If we measured every single child aged 6–59 months we would complete an exhaustive survey or census. However, imagine the huge costs in terms of money and time needed to do this. In this situation, it is much easier, cheaper and quicker to measure only a sample of the children and extrapolate the findings from this group on to the rest of the population.

B2.1.2 The importance of representative data

The representativeness of a sample is essential. Only if a sample is representative can we generalise the information we learn from the sample group to the whole population. In other words, representativeness is the prerequisite for extrapolation of results observed for the sample to the entire population.

In order for a sample to be representative of the population, the characteristics of the sample group must be similar to those of the total population. A sample that does not represent the population is 'biased'. A sample is representative if each individual or household in the population has an equal chance of being included in the sample, and the selection of one individual is independent from another individual.

Example B2.3

If we measure the nutrition status of children in a health centre in a certain village will this be representative of all the children in the village? No, probably not, as the children in the health centre are more likely to be ill and so their nutrition status will probably be worse than most of the other children in the village. The sample would probably be biased to include more malnourished children.

Example B2.4

We want to know the prevalence of malnutrition in a district. If we only measure children in villages that are near to the road will the sample represent all children in the district? No, because we have not included the children who live far away from the road. Their nutritional situation could be better or worse – we do not know. Thus, we need to include children from all over the district to ensure the sample is representative of all areas in the district. If we only measure children living near the road, our survey will be a valid description only of the nutritional situation of children living near the road.

In order for a sample not to be biased, the prevalence of malnutrition must also be relatively homogenous throughout the survey area. If the rates of malnutrition are very different in distinct parts of the survey area then the sample may not be representative of the whole population. This is discussed more fully below in Section B2.2.

B2.2 Disadvantages of sampling: the importance of choosing a sampling frame before undertaking a survey

Sampling has some disadvantages. It often does not allow disaggregation of data in the population, unless the sample was specifically designed to analyse the groups separately.

> **Example B2.5**
> If we take a sample of children from a region it would not be possible to split the results of children from each district during the analysis. Thus it would not be possible to see differences in the prevalence of malnutrition between the districts. If we need to know the prevalence by district then we must take a sample of the children in each district separately.

This means that before you design a survey you must decide those groups of people for whom you want to estimate the prevalence of malnutrition. You have to define your population, or 'sampling frame', as a first step.

If you think the prevalence of malnutrition in a particular area is higher in one group of people than another and you expect to respond to their needs differently, then you might want to undertake two separate surveys in the same area – one survey focusing on each group. For example, if there is more than one FEZ in a given district and you suspect that the prevalence of malnutrition is different in the two groups then you may need to do a separate survey for each group. Section B2.10 discusses a method for examining suspected spatial variation in the rates of malnutrition.

In some cases you might need to do more than two surveys in the same area, if there are more than two distinct population groups, but remember that surveys cost time and money. You should only conduct more than one survey if there is a real reason to suspect that there is a difference in the rate of malnutrition, and you will be able to respond to the different groups differently.

> **Example B2.6**
> You suspect that the population living in the highland FEZ of District A are worse affected by a rain failure than those living in the lowland FEZ in the same district, so you want to compare the prevalence of malnutrition in children living in the highland and lowland zones. You will need to do two separate, comparable surveys in order to do this.

However, before deciding to undertake two surveys, you need to be certain that the distinction between highland and lowland FEZ is clear and that you will be able to respond to the two groups differently. It is probable that in many areas, some farmers in the same village are classified as 'highland' farmers, but others are classified as 'lowland', and another group may have fields in both zones, so it will be difficult to decide which village belongs to which survey. Also, realistically, governments and other agencies often find it very difficult to give assistance only to some villages in a district and not others. Will the results of the survey help the authorities to target better? Is it really worthwhile undertaking two separate surveys?

Example B2.7
A new wave of refugees has just arrived in an established camp. There are now three groups of people living in and around the camp: residents, old refugees and new refugees. You think there are different rates of malnutrition in each group so you undertake three separate surveys. In this case, it would be relatively easy to separate out the three groups into three surveys. Also, it would seem logical that new refugees would need different types of assistance than the old refugees or the residents (for example, they may well need shelter, pots and pans, etc).

Note that in some cases the population group in which you are interested may be spread over more than one district. In this case it may be necessary to undertake the survey across more than one district. Before you embark on this type of survey, however, make sure you are able to respond to a problem in more than one district or that another agency is willing to do this.

B2.3 Standard error, probability and confidence intervals

A further problem with sampling is that any figures derived from a sample are subject to sampling errors because there is only partial coverage of the entire population.

Data gathered from a sample population only provide an *estimate of* the true population value. You can only obtain the true population value through exhaustive sampling (by measuring every child). Hence, whenever a sample is drawn, there is a risk that it will not be truly representative and, therefore, that the results do not reflect the true situation. Inevitably, if a second sample is drawn from the same population, slightly different results are likely to be obtained. This risk is known as the standard error. In anthropometric surveys, we generally accept a standard error of five per cent. That is to say, if a hundred sample surveys were carried out on the same population, five would give results that were not representative of the total population.

When we undertake a survey, therefore, we calculate not only an estimate of the prevalence of malnutrition but also the range of values within which the real rate of malnutrition in the entire population almost certainly lies. This range is usually called the confidence interval (see Section S5.2, Appendix S5 for more explanation). In nutrition surveys we generally accept that a 95 per cent confidence interval is appropriate (ie, with a five per cent standard error). This means we are 95 per cent certain that the true prevalence of malnutrition lies in the range given.

Example B2.8

We measure a sample of children from District A and find the prevalence of malnutrition in our sample is 9.5% and that the range, or confidence interval, around this prevalence is 7.2–12.5%. We would then say that 'the estimated prevalence of malnutrition in District A is 9.5% (95% confidence intervals are 7.2–12.5%)'. This means we are 95% certain that the actual prevalence of malnutrition in children living in District A lies between 7.2 and 12.5%.

B2.4 Essential steps in sampling

Three main sampling methods are commonly used for emergency nutrition surveys: simple random, systematic and cluster sampling. All three sampling methods use a highly ordered form of selection designed to eliminate bias.

The essential steps in obtaining a sample for any of the methods are as follows:

1. Define the population for which you need to know the estimate of malnutrition. This study population is also called the sampling frame. The sampling frame might be the children living in several villages, or a district, or a region or a refugee camp. The results you obtain from the survey will only be valid for the sampling frame as a whole. If separate estimates are needed for ethnic or geographic subgroups, or other subdivisions of the sampling frame, each of them must be treated as a separate frame for which a separate sample must be constructed (Section B2.3). Therefore, the smallest subdivision on which information is sought should be determined at the outset.

2. Obtain available population data. The best place to obtain population data for a district is usually from district government offices or other agencies working in the area. Similarly, regional level population data is usually available from regional government offices. In refugee camps you should be

able to get population data from the United Nations High Commissioner for Refugees (UNHCR) or NGOs working in the camp. If no population data are available, for example for newly displaced people or refugees, a rough population estimate should be made by counting dwellings and estimating the number of people in each dwelling.[1]

3. Choose the sampling methodology to be used. The required precision (reliability) should be identified and the necessary sample size determined accordingly.
4. Select the households or individuals to be examined.

> **Three sampling methods commonly used in emergency nutrition surveys**
>
> **Simple random sampling:** a sample base listing every individual and their location in the population is available. Individuals are randomly chosen from the list using a random number table.
>
> **Systematic sampling:** a modification of a simple random sampling that consists of picking individuals or households at regular intervals systematically, say every tenth house encountered during a house-to-house survey. There is no census list of the population, but the population is geographically concentrated and the dwellings are easy to find.
>
> **Cluster sampling:** a sampling technique that organises a population into smaller geographical areas for which the population size is estimated. Clusters are randomly selected from these geographical units according to the proportional population size. Individuals are then selected within each cluster.

B2.5 Defining the sample size

The sample size is the number of individuals to be included in the survey to represent the population of interest. Obviously, the greater number of individuals that are sampled, the more representative the sample will be. But equally, a large sample size will require more effort so it is important not to waste resources and use too big a sample.

We use standard calculations to define sample sizes. These are explained below.

---

[1] For more information, see Telford, J (1997) 'Counting and identification of beneficiary populations in emergency operations: registration and its alternatives', *RRN Good Practice Review 5*, ODI, London.

B2.5.1 Estimating sample sizes required for nutrition surveys

The sample size is the number of individuals to be included in the survey to represent the population of interest. The sample size is related to three factors:

- the expected precision. The greater the precision, or accuracy, required, the more people needed in the sample
- the expected prevalence of malnutrition. The smaller the expected proportion of children presenting with malnutrition, the smaller the size of the sample required for a given level of precision. So, as the prevalence of malnutrition approaches 50 per cent, larger sample sizes are required
- The design effect. The design effect reflects the relationship between your sampling method and the extent to which the variable which you are measuring is geographically clustered in the population. In a two-stage cluster sample we select households which are in close proximity to one another within a cluster. This means that if malnutrition itself is clustered within certain geographical locations we may end up with a sample which does not include the level of variation that exists in the sampling frame. Normally, therefore, a design effect of 2 is taken for two-stage cluster anthropometric surveys. This in effect means that the sample size is doubled (multiplied by 2) to avoid the possibility of getting a biased sample. Design effect is always 1 in simple random or systematic surveys.

In practice, the selection of sample size almost always involves a trade-off between the ideal and the feasible. A sample that is too small gives results of limited precision and, therefore, of questionable usefulness. Beyond a certain level, however, increases in sample size produce only small improvements in precision, but involve disproportionate increases in costs.

Example B2.9

A result of 10% malnutrition in a sample of 100 children would give a confidence interval ranging from approximately 4–16%, a result that cannot be interpreted usefully.

Note that a common misunderstanding about sample sizes is that the size of the sample needed for a 'good' nutrition survey is dependent on the population size. For example, people think that if your population is 10,000 then you need to sample 10% of the children. Population size only affects sample size in populations less than 5,000. The only factors which affect the sample size are those described above (see also note below in subsection B2.5.3).

B2.5.2 Software for calculating sample sizes for nutrition surveys

A piece of software for calculating sample sizes for cross-sectional surveys has recently been produced. The software (called samplexs) is available on the CD-ROM attached to this manual.[2] The programme is very easy to use. A screen like the one below pops up. You simply need to plug in the figures you expect for your survey and then press the 'calculate' button.

Example: Imagine you need to calculate a sample size calculation for a new survey. You think that the prevalence of malnutrition will be about 20%. You will use a two-stage cluster sampling method so the design effect will be about 2.0. The population size is 120,000. You will accept a result which is within +/– 5% of the true value, ie, the confidence interval is 10% wide. The screen will look like this:

The calculator shows that you need a sample size of 490 children.

---

[2] The software can also be downloaded from http://www.myatt.demon.co.uk/samplexs.htm

B2.5.3 Formulae for calculating sample sizes

You will normally use the software described above to calculate sample sizes for your survey. However, if for some reason you don't have access to this software then you should use the equations below.

$$n \ = \ k \times \frac{t^2 \times (1\text{-}p) \times p}{\varepsilon^2}$$

where:

n = sample size required

t = linked to the confidence interval required (assumed to be 1.96 in the software):

90% CI	$t = 1.62$
95% CI	$t = 1.96$
99% CI	$t = 2.57$

p = estimated prevalence of malnutrition in the population

ε = relative precision required

k = design effect (usually taken as $k = 1$ when you are undertaking a simple random survey or systematic survey, and $k = 2$ when you are undertaking a cluster survey as there are two stages in the sample design).[3]

P and ε can both be expressed either as percentages or as proportions (10% = 0.1), but both must be expressed in the same terms.

The three examples below show how the required sample size changes when the expected prevalence or precision change.

Example B2.10
Expected prevalence of malnutrition: 15%, so p = 0.15
Relative precision required (ε):   3%, so ε = 0.03
Using 95% confidence intervals t = 1.96

---

[3] A recent analysis by Save the Children UK of 66 anthropometric surveys sampled using the two-stage cluster methodology has actually found that the median design effect was 1.65. Almost 70% of all surveys had a design effect of less than 2.0. This implies that a smaller design effect than 2 would be acceptable in most situations.

For random sampling:

$$n = \frac{1.96^2 \times 0.85 \times 0.15}{0.03^2} = 544$$

For cluster sampling:

$$n = \frac{2 \times 1.96^2 \times 0.85 \times 0.15}{0.03^2} = 1088$$

Example B2.11
Expected prevalence of malnutrition: 15%, so p = 0.15
Relative precision required (ε):   1%, so ε = 0.01
Using 95% confidence intervals t = 1.96

For random sampling

$$n = \frac{1.96^2 \times 0.85 \times 0.15}{0.01^2} = 4,898$$

For cluster sampling:

$$n = \frac{2 \times 1.96^2 \times 0.85 \times 0.15}{0.01^2} = 9,796$$

Example B2.12
Expected prevalence of malnutrition: 40%, so p = 0.4
Relative precision required (ε):   3%, so ε = 0.03
Using 95% confidence intervals t = 1.96

For random sampling:

$$n = \frac{1.96^2 \times 0.6 \times 0.4}{0.03^2} = 1,024$$

For cluster sampling:

$$n = \frac{2 \times 1.96^2 \times 0.6 \times 0.4}{0.03^2} = 2,048$$

Population size

The size of the total population does not normally affect the size of the sample required. However, if the population is small and the calculated sample size turns out to be more than 10% of the total population, a correcting factor can be applied to the formula. This correction factor is used whenever the sample size is more than one tenth of the total population.[4] The revised sample size is given by the following formula:

$$\text{Revised } n_s = \frac{n}{1 + f}$$

where,

n_s = adjusted sample size for small population
n = sample size for large population (calculated as described above)
f = n/N
N = population size

Example B2.13
In example B2.10, if the total population of children aged 6–59 months was 5,000, the revised sample size for the random sampling would be:

$$\text{Revised } n = \frac{544}{1 + (544/5000)} = 491$$

B2.5.4 The importance of precision, expected prevalence and design effect

The examples in subsection B2.5.3 show the important effect on the sample size of the required precision (ε) and the expected prevalence (p). In nutrition surveys in major emergencies, the prevalence of acute malnutrition is usually 5–30 per cent, and the precision must be defined accordingly. A relative precision of around 3–5 per cent is generally appropriate. The design effect also makes a big difference to the required sample size. Table B2.1 below shows different scenarios of sample size required for varying prevalence, design effect and precision.

Currently most of the guidelines for nutrition surveys suggest using the same sample size for a cluster sample survey whatever the prevalence (ie, 30 x 30 cluster sample surveys). But, as we have seen above, the sample size varies according to the prevalence of malnutrition. You should not use a fixed sample size for all surveys. In particular, caution is required when there is a 'bad' scenario situation, ie, a high prevalence and a lot of variation between clusters leading to a large design effect, for which a large sample is needed.[5] Ideally, sample size should be determined in context.

---

[4] This correction factor is automaticaly used in sample XS software.
[5] If there is a high prevalence of oedema expected, accurate estimation of the prevalence will require a higher design effect as oedematus malnutrition is usually clustered.

Table B2.1 Different scenarios of sample size required for varying prevalence, design effect and precision

Prevalence	Precision	Sample size required		
		Design effect		
		1.5	2.0	3.0
3%	3%	186	248	372
10%	3%	576	768	1152
30%	3%	1344	1792	2689
10%	4%	324	432	648
30%	4%	756	1108	1512
30%	5%	484	645	968

Why do so many agencies standardly employ the 30 x 30 cluster methodology?

The 30 by 30 cluster methodology is based on the following assumptions:
* The prevalence of malnutrition is 50%
* The design effect is 2
* The error is 5%
* The precision is 5%

$$n = \frac{2 \times 1.96^2 \times 0.5 \times 0.5}{0.05^2} = 769$$

This gives a sample size of about 769 children. A further assumption of the method is that 15% of the data points will not be eligible (known as the non-response rate). This gives a total sample of 883 which is rounded up to 900.

Thirty clusters of thirty children are used because epidemiological studies have shown that if you have much less than 30 clusters the design effect increases and hence the survey's precision decreases. Figure B2.1 shows the mean and standard error of the relative precision of the 66 surveys recently analysed by Save the Children UK.[6] You can see that as the number of clusters increases the precision decreases. This analysis did show, however, that it is possible to use between 24 and 29 clusters and achieve precision which is not significantly different from that achieved with 30 clusters. Thus in situations where it is impossible to get 30 clusters, fewer could be taken, but unless unavoidable, this is not advised because of the risks of ending up with a non-representative result.

In fact, the assumptions made by using the 30 by 30 cluster method are not usually true. The prevalence of malnutrition is rarely 50% and the design effect

---

[6] The report by Bruce et al (2002) is on the CD-ROM attached to this manual.

Figure B2.1 Mean (and SE) of mean relative precision for all simulated samples

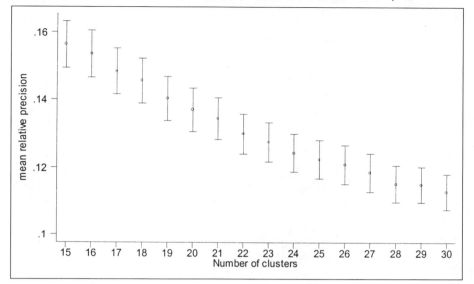

is normally less than 2.0. Moreover, the non-response rate is also usually lower than 15%. So the 30 by 30 cluster method is, in effect, the worse-case scenario method for sampling.

Some hints to help you calculate sample sizes

If you are unsure of the approximate prevalence of malnutrition, then you should look at earlier surveys from the same area. If there are no prior survey data available then you should err towards assuming higher prevalence, which will result in a bigger sample and hence put you on the safe side.

The same is true when you are estimating the potential design effect in a cluster survey. In this situation you need to see if there is any information on the design effect in the past. If you cannot find any information on this then assume that the design effect is 2 if you are using the two-stage cluster methodology.

When thinking about how many clusters to choose when you have a sample size less than 900, one important rule of thumb is that it is more important to keep the number of clusters relatively high (30 or more) and decrease the number of children per cluster rather than decrease the number of clusters. In practice, this means that if you only need 800 children in a survey then you should still use 30 clusters but only measure 800/30 (= 26) children per cluster.

B2.6 Simple random sampling

Simple random sampling is the best method – when it can be used – because you can measure fewer children and so it is quicker. An up-to-date list of all individuals or households in the population is required, with enough information to allow them to be located. Individuals are randomly chosen by (a) picking them out of a hat, or (b) using a random number table (see Section S5.3, Appendix S5).

> **Example B2.14**
> Simple random sampling might be useful if you go to a place where all the names of the children are known and recorded, for example, a health centre where every child is registered. You could give each child a number and draw as many numbers out of the hat as you need. You could then call each child to be measured and/or interviewed.

In practice, in many rural areas of the developing world, a reliable population list is rarely available, and it is sometimes practical to use the following alternative procedure:

1. Determine the sample size (the number of children required) as shown in Section B2.5. Assume that the sample required is 544 for the rest of this example.
2. Go to the area and make a list of all households[7] with children aged 6–59 months.
3. Assign each household on the list an identification number.
4. Determine the required number of households. The first step is to calculate the average number of children in each household. This figure is equal to the total number of children divided by the number of households: 10,000/11,000 = 0.9. Therefore, we need to visit 604 households (544/0.9) to complete the sample.
5. Select 604 households using a random number table. Alternatively pick household identification numbers out of a hat or plastic bag (if this type of selection is done in public the community can see how households are selected).

---

[7] It is important to carefully define a household: one person who lives alone or a group of persons, related or unrelated, who share food or make common provisions for food and possibly other essentials for living; the smallest and most common unit of production, consumption and organisation in societies. Polygamous households are sometimes several households and are sometimes one household.

6. Visit all the households whose numbers were drawn. Do not visit any other households. No households should be substituted for any reason. In a nutritional survey, all children in the specified age group belonging to each of the selected households must be measured. This means if there is more than one eligible child in a household they should all be included in the survey.[8] If a child is not present at the time of the survey go back to the house later to find the child (you should continue to look for the missing children until you have to leave the survey area).

B2.7 Systematic sampling

Systematic sampling eliminates the need for complete, up-to-date population data. But you need a relatively small geographic area, a reasonably accurate plan

Figure B2.2 Example of a community where systematic sampling is possible (Source: Médecins Sans Frontières, in press)

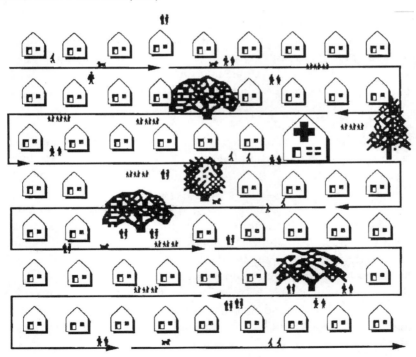

---

[8] Some agencies recommend only measuring one eligible child per household (if there is more than one child then one of them is randomly selected for measuring). However, this method has been shown to result in a biased sample and hence has been discredited (see section B2.9). Always measure all the children aged 6–59 months in each selected household.

or map showing *all* households; and an orderly layout, or site plan, which makes it possible to go systematically through the whole site.

The procedure is as follows:

1. Determine the sample size (the number of children required) as shown in Section B2.5. Assume that the sample required is 544 for the rest of this example.
2. Obtain a map of the site and trace a continuous route on the map, which passes in front of every household.
3. Determine the number of inhabitants and the number of households (let us assume 50,000 people and 11,000 households as an example).
4. Determine the number of children aged 6–59 months in the population. The proportion of children in this age group is usually quite stable, around 20 per cent. However, in certain situations, when high mortality is suspected, the proportion can be smaller. In this case, the proportion of children can be estimated from a rapid survey covering 30 households at random. (In our example, assuming the proportion of children aged 6–59 months is 20 per cent, we have 10,000 children.)
5. Determine the required number of households.
6. Determine the 'sampling interval' by dividing the total number of households by the number that must be visited. In our example, if the total number of households is 11,000, the sample interval = 11,000/604 = 18.2. You should round down to the nearest whole number, therefore one household in every 18 should be visited.
7. Select the first household to be visited. The first household is randomly selected within the sampling interval (1–18) by drawing a random number which is smaller than the sampling interval (see Section S6.4, Appendix S6 for more explanation). Assume the number drawn is '5', so start with the fifth house.
8. Select the next household by adding the sampling interval to the first household selected (or counting the number of households along the prescribed route), for example, 5+18 = 23. Continue in this way (for example, visit houses 5, 23, 41, 59, etc) until the number of households required for the survey has been systematically selected.
9. Measure all children aged 6–59 months in the selected households. If two eligible children are found in a household include both. If no children are found in a house, go to the next house in the sample (by adding the sampling interval again). For example, if there are no children in house 23, then go to house 41 and continue looking for children there.
10. If a child is not present at the time of the survey go back to the house later to find the child (you should continue to look for the missing children until you leave the survey area). If you do not get enough children and you have

finished going to all the houses you had planned to, then you should find a new sampling interval and start the process again until you have got enough children. For example, if you need another 40 children then you should find a new sampling interval: 11,000/40 = 275. You now need to visit every 275th household to find the remaining children.

It is important not to overestimate the proportion of children aged 6–59 months when calculating the sampling interval. If you do this the sampling interval will be too large and the total number of children measured will not be enough.

B2.8 Two-stage cluster sampling

Two-stage cluster sampling is used in large populations, where no accurate population register is available and households cannot be visited systematically. This is very common in rural populations in the developing world and so this method is the most commonly used in emergency assessments. Another advantage of cluster sampling is that it is more convenient than simple random sampling, because a cluster design reduces the distance travelled by the survey team. The number of sites visited is equal to the number of clusters, unlike simple random sampling where every child could be located in a different place or site. The sampling is split into two stages:

Stage one clusters, or sampling sites, within the total population are selected randomly according to their size.

Stage two an appropriate number of children are randomly selected within each selected cluster.

This two-stage process is applied separately to each population of interest – for each sampling frame. For example, if we need to know the prevalence of malnutrition for separate districts, then we need to do this twice – once for each district.

The larger the number of clusters, the higher the probability that the sample will be truly representative of the population because more sites will be studied (see Section B2.5). This means that the more clusters there are, the smaller the confidence interval will be around the estimate of the prevalence of malnutrition and the more accurate the estimate of malnutrition will be. In practice, physical constraints will limit the number of children that can conveniently be measured in a cluster and the number of clusters (or sites) that can be visited.

Very often a 30 x 30 two-stage cluster sampling method is used in emergency nutrition assessments. This means measuring 30 children in each of 30 clusters (900 children in total). This pattern of sampling has been adopted by many

Figure B2.3 Example of a community where two-stage cluster sampling is needed

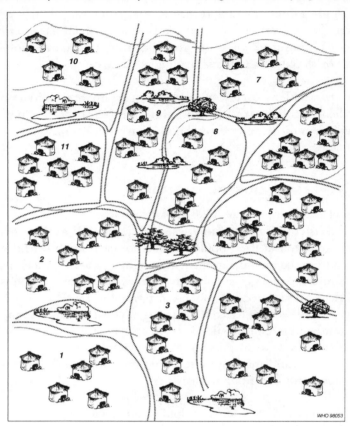

agencies because the sample size allows for a worst-case scenario in terms of the malnutrition prevalence and design effect (see Section B2.5). However, it is often not necessary to measure as many children as this if, for example, the prevalence of malnutrition is less. Sometimes it is necessary to take more than 30 clusters in a survey (see Section B2.9). Remember that you should always determine your required sample size for each nutrition survey to make sure resources are not wasted.

B2.8.1 Stage one: selecting the cluster

The basic principle of this first stage (cluster selection) is that the relative size of a locality[9] will affect the chance of it being included the survey. This is called

---

[9] Note that the term locality refers either to a village or some other small administrative unit in this chapter.

probability proportional to size (PPS) sampling. Localities are allocated random numbers in proportion to their relative population size. This requires the grouping of the population into smaller geographical units (localities). The smallest available geographical unit is always chosen, as long as population data is available. So if village data are available, use these localities as the geographical unit. If village data are not available, use district-level data. If there are no population data, draw a map of the area and roughly divide the area into sections (localities) of about equal size, following as far as possible existing geographic or administrative boundaries (see figure B2.3). Each section should have at least 300 inhabitants.

Then follow this procedure:

1. Determine the sample size (the number of children required) using the methods described in Section B2.5. Assume that the sample will be 30 clusters of 30 children for the rest of this example.

2. Obtain the best available population data for each locality. This is usually obtained from the local government offices. In a stable population, such as a drought-affected region with little in- and out-migration, a census that is several years old may still be acceptable as a basis for population proportionate sampling. However, in refugee situations where influx continues, reliable up-to-date counts are important for a valid sample. Alternatively, if no population data are available then you can estimate the relative size of the population living in each section of the map with a key informant (see subsection B2.9.5 for more details).

3. Obtain the best available data about the number of under-fives in each village. In most circumstances, the total population rather than the population of children under five can be used to develop the sampling frame, since children form a relatively stable fraction of the population and the total population figures are usually easier to obtain. However, if you know that the proportion of under-fives varies from area to area, you should try to collect accurate data on this.

4. Next, make a table with six columns (see below). The first column should include the name of each locality (for example, village, district or section on map). These names can be in any order. The second column should contain the estimated total population of each unit. The third column should contain the estimated population of the children in each unit.

Geographical unit	Estimated total population	Estimated children 6–59 months	Cumulative population 6–59 months	Attributed numbers	Location of clusters
Locality 1	2,500	500			
Locality 2	1,000	200			
Locality 3	800	160			
Locality 4	3,250	650			
Etc …	…	…			
…	…	…			
Total	50,000	10,000			

5. Next add two more columns. The fourth column should contain the cumulative population of the children (obtained by adding the population of each unit to the combined population figure of the preceding units). The fifth column should contain the attributed numbers for each unit – the range of the cumulative population for each unit.

Geographical unit	Estimated total population	Estimated children 6–59 months	Cumulative population 6–59 months	Attributed numbers	Location of clusters
Locality 1	2,500	500	500	1–500	
Locality 2	1,000	200	700	501–700	
Locality 3	800	160	860	701–860	
Locality 4	3,250	650	1,610	861–1,610	
Etc …	…	…		1,611– …	
…	…	…			
			10,000	… –10,000	
Total	50,000	10,000			

6. Calculate the 'sampling interval'. In cluster sampling, the sampling interval is obtained by dividing the 6–59 months population by the desired number of clusters, which is usually 30. In this example, the sampling interval is 10,000/30 = 333.
7. Determine the location of the first cluster. Its location is randomly chosen by selecting a number within the first sampling interval (1–333 in this example). The number can be randomly selected using a random number table, etc (see Section S5.3, Appendix S5 for further explanation). Let us assume that we chose 256 as our starting point. This number places the first cluster in 'Locality 1' in our example because it has the attributed numbers 1–500.
8. Select the other clusters. Add the sampling interval sequentially to the starting number until 30 numbers are chosen. Each number chosen represents the population of a geographic unit. In this example, the first cluster is at 256

(Locality 1), the second cluster at 256 + 333 = 589 (Locality 2), the third cluster is at 589 + 333 = 922 (Locality 4), the fourth cluster is at 922 + 333 = 1,255 (Locality 4), etc. A large geographical unit may appear twice – two clusters are drawn in Locality 4 in our example. In the same way, a small geographical unit (smaller than the sampling interval) may not be selected – Locality 3 in our example.

Geographical unit	Estimated total population	Estimated children 6–59 months	Cumulative population 6–59 months	Attributed numbers	Location of clusters
Locality 1	2,500	500	500	1–500	1
Locality 2	1,000	200	700	501–700	1
Locality 3	800	160	860	701–860	0
Locality 4	3,250	650	1,610	861–1,610	2
Etc ...	...	...		1,611– ...	...
...	...	...	...	...	...
			10,000	... –10,000	
Total	50,000	10,000			30

Remember: never change a sampling site because it is too remote. If an area is too remote it should not be included in the sampling frame from the beginning. (This should be recorded in the assessment report.)

B2.8.2 Stage two: selection of children in the clusters

Having identified the 30 clusters, a team of data collectors should go to the site of each cluster. Let us assume that we obtained locality level population data and have arrived at one of the selected localities.

At any given cluster, or locality, once discussions have been held with the local leader(s), the following procedure should be followed:

1. Go to the centre of the selected locality (ask local people for information).
2. Randomly choose a direction by spinning a pencil or pen on the ground and noting the direction in which it points when it stops.
3. Walk in the direction indicated by the pen, from the centre to the outer perimeter of the locality, counting the number of households along this line.[10]
4. Select the first household to be visited by drawing a random number between one and the number of households counted when walking. For example, if the number of households counted was 27, then select a random number

---

[10] If the distances are too big to do this you should divide the cluster up into smaller units. A unit should be randomly selected and the survey should begin in the centre of the unit.

1–27. If the number five was chosen, then the fifth household on the walking line is the first you should visit.

5. Go to the first household and examine *all* children aged 6–59 months in the household.

6. The subsequent households are chosen by proximity. In a locality where there is a high population concentration, proceed by always choosing the next house to the right or to the left (decide which at the beginning of the survey and stick to it). Continue to go to the left/right until the required number of children has been measured. The same method should be used for all clusters. However, if the locality has a very spread-out population, then proceed by simply choosing the nearest house. The nearest house is the one with the door nearest to the last house surveyed, whether it is on the right or left (this should save you a lot of time in an area where the dwellings are very spread out). Continue the process until the required number of children has been measured.

7. If there are no children under five in a household proceed to the next house.

8. All eligible children are included and thus should be measured and weighed. This means that all children in the last house should be measured even if this means exceeding the number required. If a child is not present at the time of the survey go back to the house later to find the child (you should continue to look for the missing children until you leave the survey area). If you cannot find a child then you need to replace it with another by continuing the sampling methodology. If a child has been admitted to a feeding centre, the team must go to the centre and measure him or her there.

It is extremely important to follow this house-to-house method of selecting children if you are undertaking a survey. If you just called for children to be brought to the centre of the locality, it is likely that some of the children could be missed. This could result in bias. In addition to preventing bias, the house-to-house method also allows you to administer household questionnaires at someone's home.

9. If you run out of houses to measure in a locality and have not found sufficient children (that is, you have not found 30 children) then you should proceed to the nearest locality. When you arrive at the nearest locality you should repeat the process of spinning a pen and randomly selecting a house to start at (steps 1–8 described above). Proceed from house to house until you have measured sufficient children.

10. If a child is not present at the time of the survey go back to the house later to find the child (you should continue to look for the missing children until you leave the survey area).

Note that sometimes you will draw more than one cluster from the same locality if the locality is very large. In this situation, you should 'segment and sample'. This means roughly splitting the community into two equal parts (you can get advice from local residents for this) and then take a cluster from each of the parts. This would mean repeating steps 1–8 for each section of the community separately.

Biases encountered by calling children to the centre of a locality
If you call for children to come to the centre of the locality to be measured, many different types of bias can occur:
- smaller children, who can be more easily carried, may be brought
- older children may be more likely to come, as they will be curious about what is going on
- sick, weak and most malnourished children may be left at home if the mother does not want to disturb them
- if there is supplementary food only for the most severely malnourished then only these children may be brought.

You cannot tell which type of bias will happen when you call children to the centre of locality, therefore you must go from house to house to find children.

It should be noted that cluster sampling does not completely fulfil the requirements of a representative sample. This is because several children are selected within a cluster by proximity and therefore the choice of a child is not independent from the choice of other children. Within each cluster, children will have a tendency to be similar as far as nutritional status is concerned. This phenomenon is called the 'design effect'. The design effect is taken into account when calculating the sample size (see Section B2.5).

B2.9 Avoiding sampling bias

There are three points at which sampling bias can be introduced:

1) Bias in the sampling frame
This can occur if the information about the sampling frame is inaccurate or out of date. Two-stage cluster sampling relies on sampling clusters from locations according to their relative size. If the population data is very inaccurate. this can mean that underpopulated areas are oversampled and vice versa. This can be avoided by using a relative rather than absolute size estimate (see subsection B2.9.5).

A very common source of bias occurs when a population which is not representative of the sampling frame is sampled. For example, in southern Sudan anthropometric surveys are conducted in payams (the equivalent of sub-districts). In these surveys, only clusters within a certain distance of the airstrip are eligible for inclusion. However, results are usually presented as representative of the whole payam. In this situation, if for security reasons the whole area cannot be sampled then the results should be presented as representing the situation only in the communities within a certain radius of the airstrip. The report could also discuss whether the situation was expected to be better or worse among these communities as compared with the rest of the payam.

2) Household selection bias

Household selection bias can be introduced when the rules for sampling are not strictly followed in two-stage cluster sampling. The first common example of when household selection bias is introduced is when surveyors arrive at a cluster and immediately spin the bottle and start sampling households from the centre of the cluster. They have missed out the essential step of walking to the edge of the cluster, counting the households in order to randomly select the starting point. People who live in the centre of villages and towns are likely to be wealthier than households on the periphery. If only children from this type of household are included in the survey the results will be biased. This should be avoided by carefully following the sampling rules.

Another common mistake is to only visit households with children under five for the mortality survey. This generally occurs when anthropometric and mortality surveys are done simultaneously and by the same team. This means that households which have recently lost a child under five years but have no other children under five will be excluded and the results will probably underestimate the true under-five mortality rate. The crude mortality rate will also be very biased by only visiting these households (see also Section C2.2.5).

3) Child selection bias

Age and sex biases can be introduced if children who are not in the household at the time of the survey are not ultimately included. For this reason it is very important that you return to households to measure children who were absent.

Child selection bias is also commonly introduced when only one child, rather than all children 6–59 months, is included in the sample. This results in under-representation of children in the sample who have siblings under five. In many places children in families with more young children are likely to have worse nutritional status, as there are more children to share similar resources in bigger families. Therefore, if there are fewer of these children in the sample than really exist in the population, you will underestimate the prevalence of malnutrition. Another common mistake occurs when households are not actually visited and community members are asked to bring children to a central point in the village for measurement. This can result in significant bias but it is not easy to judge the direction of bias (see box above). The only way to avoid these biases is to follow the sampling rules very carefully.

Child selection bias is discussed further in subsection B3.4.2, where it is recommended that you check to see whether there are age and sex biases in the sampling.

B2.10 Common constraints of cluster sampling in rural populations

This section will describe some common constraints encountered when using the cluster sampling technique in rural populations. Suggestions for how to overcome the constraints are also given.

B2.10.1 Population scattered over a large area

This is a very common phenomenon, particularly in pastoral areas. Allow more time for travelling between sites. Perhaps select more clusters (say 35) and a small number of children per cluster, to ensure that the same number can be found in each site to prevent bias.

> **Example B2.15**
> You want to undertake a cluster survey and have calculated that you need 900 children. The survey is going to be in a pastoralist area and you have heard that the population lives in very small settlements, often with only 25 households in each locality. So, you decide to select 35 clusters and will measure 25 children in each cluster. This will still give you a good estimate of the prevalence of mal-nutrition (with small confidence intervals), but will probably be more time-consuming than undertaking 30 clusters, as you will have to travel to more sites. If the villages were even smaller then you could consider undertaking 50 clusters with 18 children in them.

In some situations where the population is very spread out you may deliberately choose to undertake a survey without sampling certain sections of the population. You might chose to sample only the population that lives together in larger settlements, which would save you the time and money needed to get out to the more scattered population. This would mean not including the population estimates from the scattered area when you are originally selecting your sample (as described in Section B2.8.1). If this is the case, you must remember to describe who you excluded from the sampling frame in your report of the survey. You might also want to discuss what the nutritional situation is like in the areas you did not sample (if you have any information on this).

B2.10.2 Population is very mobile

If you are attempting to undertake a survey in an area where the population frequently moves large distances, then it likely you may arrive at a cluster and find there is no one there and no one nearby. If you suspect this might happen, you should select some extra clusters before you start the survey, so that if one cluster is deserted you can replace it with another one. Do this by selecting more than 30 clusters (say 33) right at the beginning of the sampling (see Section B2.8.1). You should plan to survey all 33 clusters. If, however, it is not possible to survey one or more of them, there should still be at least 30 that have been surveyed. It is worth noting here that 30 clusters is the number determined by statisticians to be the best balance between representativeness and workload. Undertaking any more than 30 clusters results in a minimal improvement in representativeness and considerable extra workload, so you should undertake 33 clusters only if really necessary.

B2.10.3 Limited access to some areas because of insecurity or inadequate roads

If access is completely impossible, then a sample of the area cannot be taken. The alternative is to take a sample of people who have recently left the area – eg, to find people at a food distribution or health clinic, or a market day. If displaced people are arriving from a certain area then it's possible to assess them as they arrive, giving an indication of what the rate of malnutrition is in the area they have left. This type of surveying will give you a biased (unrepresentative) sample, and only a very rough indication of the true picture.

If access is possible only in some areas, you might choose just to draw your sample from the secure areas. This would mean not including the population estimates from the insecure area when you are originally selecting your sample (as described in Section B2.8.1). If this is the case, you must remember to describe who you excluded from the sampling frame in your report of the survey. You might also want to discuss what the nutritional situation is like in the areas you did not sample (if you have any information on this).

Example B2.16

You want to undertake a cluster survey in a district with 30 villages, but you know that three of the villages are very insecure and you do not want to send your team into those areas. Instead, you decide only to draw your 30 clusters from the 27 secure villages. Thus you will only sum the cumulative frequency of the population from the 27 villages. In your survey report you will be sure to mention that the results are only representative for the 27 villages.

Alternatively, if access is possible only in some areas, then you may want to do purposive sampling (see Section B2.10). This means you will only be selecting representative localities from certain areas before you start the survey. Remember to report that your sample will not be representative of the whole area.

B2.10.4 Variation in the rate of malnutrition is suspected

A cluster survey of the entire area will give you a single estimate of the prevalence of malnutrition and will not show you the differences within the area. Divide the area into smaller sections, according to where you think the differences are, and select 30 clusters from each of those areas. Alternatively, undertake purposive sampling of each different area (see Section B2.10).

B2.10.5 No reliable data on population size

Use as many sources of information as possible to list all the known villages in the area to be surveyed. Estimate the relative size, based on local knowledge, and assign a relative score to each location (very big = 5, big = 4, medium = 3, small = 2, very small = 1). Use these estimates to select the required number of clusters using PPS sampling.

B2.11 Purposive sampling

The simple random, systematic and two-stage cluster methods of sampling assume that the rate of malnutrition is similar throughout the area to be surveyed. This may not always be true and you may need to know the level of malnutrition in more geographically specific areas. You may need this information when:

- you think rates of malnutrition are patchy and not uniform – eg, if certain areas have been cut off from markets and trade due to insecurity you might expect their rates of malnutrition to be higher
- you would like to validate your conclusions about the major causes of malnutrition (see Part A) or the most nutritionally vulnerable areas. You may have conducted an anthropometric survey but in your causal analysis you indicate a belief that some parts of the area covered by the survey are likely to be worse off than others, so you may wish to investigate further
- you need to prioritise your intervention. You may have found from the anthropometric survey that rates of malnutrition are very high and your causal analysis has concluded that a feeding programme would be the most appropriate short-term intervention. You cannot, however, cover the whole area with a feeding programme immediately. You need to know in which

areas you should start operations or in which areas you should locate inpatient feeding centres. Of course, the location of feeding or distribution points is based not only on the prevalence of malnutrition in the immediate vicinity but also on other factors that might be important – eg, logistics and the existence of health facilities.

Under no circumstances should you try to look at the prevalence of malnutrition in each cluster of a survey dataset in order to shed light on the level of malnutrition in specific geographical areas. The cluster is not representative and could well give you a false picture.

In purposive sampling you are deliberately selecting sites where you will measure children. These sites are representative of certain areas, whereas when you use the other sampling methods, the sites at which you measure are decided either by chance (simple random and systematic) or according to their relative population size (cluster sampling). Prevalance of malnutrition may then be estimated for each village, but it will not be statistically valid to use the figures obtained to make estimates for the area as a whole.

Example B2.17 describes a case where purposive sampling, followed by exhaustive or systematic sampling, was conducted in order to prioritise locations for food distribution.

Example B2.17

You are planning a targeted supplementary feeding programme for malnourished young children in response to a food crisis in Fik Zone, Somali Region of Ethiopia. You know that there are different concentrations of displaced and resident children throughout the zone, but you do not know the exact distribution of the displaced. You think the children of displaced people are more vulnerable to malnutrition than the residents' children, but you want to include both displaced and resident children who are malnourished in your programme. You are trying to work out how much food to send to which area, but it is difficult to know which areas are most affected and where most of the malnourished children are. In order to estimate where you will need the most food

(where most of the malnourished children are) you could undertake some purposive sampling. Make a list of the localities or areas that you think have similar conditions (eg, Bernil, Dihun and possibly Hamero as shown in the table). Undertake exhaustive or systematic sampling (for which a sample size has to be calculated, as in Section B2.5) in one or two of the representative towns/areas (in this instance Bernil). Then decide what interventions may be needed in the area. Your results may look something like this.

Site	Estimated rate of malnutrition in each site	Other locations where conditions are thought to be similar
Bernil	25%	Dihun, possibly Hamero
Garasley	15%	Fik, Segeg, Dundumad, possibly Hamero, Gerinka
Gasangas	40%	Ayun

From these results you could decide that Gasnagas and Ayun were the priority areas for food distributions.

When purposive sampling is conducted, areas are chosen because they represent a certain situation rather than the situation of the whole population. However, it is important that the choice of areas is based on a sound understanding of the situation to avoid misleading results.

Example B2.18
Save the Children UK undertook anthropometric surveys in each of five separate food economy zones (FEZs) in North Darfur, Sudan, all conducted by well-trained teams and implemented according to internationally recognised standards. Detailed food economy and food security data stretching back over ten years, including historical records of market prices, terms of trade, harvests, and other sources of income, supplemented the data from these surveys, provided a baseline and enabled the cross-sectional nutritional data to be set in context. The results were very worrying: an average of 24% global malnutrition, six months to the next harvest and clear signs that coping capacities had been exhausted.

Shortly afterwards another assessment consisted of a team of three people visiting 27 locations. The team held meetings with the local authorities, visited the health facilities and water points, held discussions with families and screened under-five children using MUAC measurements taken via purposive samples from groups thought to be at high risk (eg, displaced). The team systematically tried to focus its attention on the most vulnerable areas and families with the aim of describing the situation of the most at-risk rather than giving a general picture of the situation. Given their attempts to focus on the most vulnerable their results were surprising. Of the 424 children that they measured, only 1% had a MUAC <110mm, 5% had between 110mm and 125mm and 12.5% between 126mm and 135mm. A very different picture from the results of the Save the Children UK surveys. A likely explanation for these differences is that the assumption that the displaced are the most vulnerable was false. In Darfur, this assumption was an oversimplification, as the displaced living around the wadis are those who still have cattle remaining, and are in fact the richest segment of the population.

Systematic and exhaustive sampling of areas which have been purposively selected can be very time-consuming if the community is large. An alternative is Acceptance Sampling. This requires a much smaller sample size (usually fewer than 50 children) and allows conclusions to be drawn as to whether the situation in the community is bad or good. Bad or good are defined before the sampling according to the level of malnutrition deemed to be serious or satisfactory. Acceptance sampling takes 4–5 hours per community (Myatt et al, 2003). A detailed description of how the sample size can be calculated and how the sampling is conducted is given in a manual on the CD-ROM attached to this manual.

Example B2.19
Save the Children in Kinshasa wanted to assess the rates of malnutrition but knew it was highly likely that rates of malnutrition would vary substantially between different areas of the city. The team therefore used secondary data and their personal knowledge to construct a map with the areas marked as good or bad depending on their judgement of how much malnutrition they expected. Kikimi zone was selected as representative of some of the bad areas and LQAS (Lot Quality Assurance Sampling), which is a type of acceptance sampling, was conducted to assess the level of malnutrition; 21 children were measured. Nine children were found to be malnourished (<80% weight for height or oedema). These results allowed us to conclude with 90% confidence that the situation was not good (ie, good was defined as acute malnutrition <5%) and 81% confidence that the situation was bad (ie, bad was defined as acute malnutrition >15%). A feeding centre was subsequently located in this zone.

B2.12 Cross-sectional and longitudinal sampling

Cross-sectional data are used to describe the nutritional situation of a population at a given point in time. The results of cross-sectional nutrition assessments are often used to compare the nutritional situation of one population with another. However, for nutrition assessments to be comparable they must use representative samples.

Example B2.20
NGOs, governments and donors compare the results of nutrition surveys undertaken using the same methodologies in different places to see which areas are the worst affected. This assists all the agencies in targeting limited resources to beneficiaries most in need. If the surveys are conducted using different sampling methods, for example, purposive and cluster, it may not be possible to compare them.

Sometimes we might want to assess the nutritional situation of a population over time to see if the situation is improving or deteriorating, or if there are seasonal differences in nutritional status (see Chapter A1). There are two ways to do this:

- by repeating cross-sectional surveys
- by undertaking longitudinal surveys.[11]

The sampling methods described in this chapter can be used to obtain cross-sectional data. To show longer-term changes (for example, seasonal changes) you would repeat the sampling procedure and survey on the same population some months, or years, after the original survey. The individuals or clusters in the sample may be different in the second survey, as they are chosen randomly and so will probably not be the same. However, the two surveys will be directly comparable if the same methodology is used and therefore the results can be analysed to look for differences over time. The procedure to compare two sets of survey results is described in Chapter D1.

Summary

- Samples are taken to save time and resources.
- If a sample is unrepresentative or biased, the results of a survey cannot be generalised to the whole population.
- All sampling methods use a highly ordered form of selection designed to eliminate bias.
- Under normal circumstances, emergency nutrition assessments should employ either simple random, systematic or two-stage cluster sampling methods.
- Sample size calculations should be made for every nutrition assessment in order to reduce wasting resources.
- In certain circumstances, it may be necessary to make adjustments to the standard sampling methodology. This is acceptable, as long as it is clearly described in the assessment report. Remember that inappropriate changes to survey methods are liable to give misleading results.

---

[11] Longitudinal surveys involve measuring the same children regularly. Describing this type of survey is beyond the scope of this manual.

Chapter B3
Analysis of anthropometric results

In order to compare easily the results of different anthropometric surveys, we need to present the results in a standardised format. This means the analysis of the data collected also has to be conducted in a standardised way. This chapter will describe a standard analysis of results, including:

- data preparation and cleaning
- sample description
- analysis of anthropometric and morbidity data.

Model results tables will also be explained. Further discussion will focus on analysing other data commonly collected during anthropometric surveys – eg, vaccination coverage.

B3.1 Analysis by computer or by hand?

The analysis presented in this chapter will assume that you do not have a computer and the software available for computing anthropometric data. In fact, a computer software program called EpiInfo is freely available and is provided on the CD-ROM attached to this manual: version 6.04b is recommended. The Centers for Disease Control and Prevention (CDC) specifically designed this program to analyse public health data. A second program, Epinut, was then designed to analyse anthropometric survey data. EpiInfo and Epinut can calculate all the nutritional indices from age, weight, height and sex data.

Save the Children UK has developed a user manual for EpiInfo and Epinut, which is also available on the CD-ROM attached to this manual. The manual describes how to analyse anthropometric survey data using the program. Unfortunately, it takes time to learn the Epinut and EpiInfo programs. This chapter will only describe calculations that are possible by hand.

B3.2 Calculating nutrition indices for each child

To analyse nutrition survey data you need to calculate the WHM and WHZ for every child in the dataset. The equations to calculate WHM and WHZ are given below (see Chapter B1 for a more detailed explanation).

$$\text{WHM} = \frac{\text{individual's weight} \times 100}{\text{median reference weight}}$$

$$\text{WHZ} = \frac{\text{individual's weight} - \text{median reference weight}}{\text{standard deviation of weight for the reference population}}$$

WHMs are often calculated at the time of the survey (see Section S6.1, Appendix S6 for a model anthropometric questionnaire). However, it may be more difficult to calculate z-scores in the field. These should probably be calculated either at night, or after the survey (when a chair, table and good light are available). When you have finished calculating WHM and WHZ for each child, your anthropometry form should look something like the one shown in Table B3.1.

B3.3 Data preparation and cleaning

Before starting the analysis, the data needs to be prepared and 'cleaned'. Some of the information you have collected during the survey will probably be incorrect. This is because each child's record has undergone a process of measurement, interview, interpretation, listening and recording. Mistakes can be made during any of these processes. Examples of common mistakes include:

- reply error (incorrect information heard)
- data recording error
- measurement error.

If any of these mistakes occur then the information you have on your record sheets will not be 'true' information. The objective of data preparation and cleaning is to remove this 'false' data so that the data we actually analyse and report are real.

When we check the data during the analysis we have to look for pieces of data that are either missing, out of our required range, or extreme.

B3.3.1 Missing data

If your survey records of a child are missing certain pieces of information then it will not be possible to include that child in all the analyses of the anthropometric data. Of course, some pieces of information are more critical than others. The list below shows which analyses you can't undertake when you are missing different types of data:

Table B3.1 Nutrition survey: anthropometric data

Survey district: 011   Village: Worset   Cluster Number: 12

Date: 21/6/93   Team Number: 3

HH No.	Child No.	Name	Age in months	Sex (F/M)	Oedema (Y/N)	Weight (kg) ± 100g	Height (cm) ±0.1cm	WHM	Vaccination BCG mark (Y/N)	Measles Card = 1 (Yes but no card = 2 No = 0)	Vit A (Y/N/DK)	WHZ
1	1	Belay Endris	49	F	N	12.9	96.5	89.1	N	1	Y	-1.24
1	2	Alem Endris	18	F	N	8.2	74.5	86.5	N	1	N	-1.51
2	3	Zeyneba Alebachew	41	F	N	10.9	92.5	80.7	Y	2	Y	-2.20
3	4	Toyba Aragaw	50	F	N	12.3	95.5	86.5	N	1	N	-1.54
3	5	Mohmmed Aragaw	13	M	N	5.7	65.5	78.5	Y	1	N	-2.19
5	6	Meka Endris	54	F	Y	15.7	104.5	94.6	N	0	N	-0.61
6	7	Asya Hussen	28	F	N	10.7	87.0	87.2	N	0	Y	-1.43
13	8	Mersha Said	36	F	N	10.8	87.5	88.8	N	0	Y	-1.25
15	9	Endris Yimer	50	M	N	13.6	102.5	82.8	N	2	Y	-1.98
15	10	Awol Yimer	18	M	N	8.8	77.5	84.8	N	2	N	-1.90
16	11	Ketemaw Abitew	24	M	N	6.9	76.5	67.4	Y	0	N	-3.31
17	12	Said Yimer	39	M	N	12.9	93.0	92.3	N	2	N	-0.88
19	13	Fatima Said	15	F	N	8.1	73.0	88.6	N	0	Y	-1.25
20	14	Aleme Adem	50	F	N	15.9	105.0	95.0	N	0	Y	-0.57
20	15	Habtamu Adem	30	M	N	12.7	91.0	94.1	Y	0	N	-0.67
21	16	Ebre Girma	23	M	N	9.9	83.0	86.0	N	1	N	-1.82

HH No.	Child No.	Name	Age in months	Sex (F/M)	Oedema (Y/N)	Weight (kg) ± 100g	Height (cm) ±0.1cm	WHM	Vaccination BCG mark (Y/N)	Measles Card = 1 Yes but no card = 2 No = 0	Vit A (Y/N)	WHZ
22	17	Ahmed Said	19	M	N	7.6	79.0	71.0	Y	0	N	-3.66
23	18	Ali Mekonen	43	M	N	14.8	100.5	93.2	N	2	Y	-0.78
27	19	Moh'd Ahmed	45	M	N	14.5	94.0	102.0	Y	2	Y	0.19
28	20	Rukya Endri	45	F	N	15.6	103.0	96.4	Y	1	Y	-0.40
28	21	Aregu Endri	30	F	N	10.3	83.0	90.2	Y	1	Y	-1.06
29	22	Zemal Yimam	38	M	N	11.2	89.0	86.0	N	2	Y	-1.59
30	23	Ebrahim Said	46	M	N	15.3	98.5	99.7	N	2	Y	-0.04
31	24	Merima Kassaw	18	F	N	7.2	69.0	89.0	N	1	Y	-1.16
32	25	Nurye Jemal	50	M	Y	13.5	98.5	87.9	N	1	Y	-1.38
32	26	Shikur Jemal	48	F	N	10.7	91.5	80.6	N	1	N	-2.21
33	27	Ali Ahmed	46	M	N	13.1	95.5	89.8	N	2	Y	-1.17
33	28	Addisu Ahmed	19	M	N	9.8	80.5	88.9	N	2	N	-1.40
34	29	Adane Yimmer	23	M	N	7.9	77.5	75.5	N	1	N	-2.53
34	30	Tayech Tesfaye	58	M	N	11.5	100.0	74.8	N	1	N	-2.85

HH = household

- Oedema: if the child's data on oedema is missing then you cannot include her/him in any of the anthropometric analyses.
- Age: if the child's information on age is missing you can still include her/him in the assessment of wasting because the index does not require age. However, you would need to be sure that s/he is eligible to be in the survey, ie, that s/he is between 6 and 59 months old or less than 110cm.
- Sex: if information on the child's sex is missing you cannot include her/him in the assessment of wasting because the reference population information on height and weight is sex specific. S/he can, of course, still be included in an analysis of oedema because any child with oedema is severely malnourished.
- Height: if the child's information on height is missing you cannot include her/him in the assessment of wasting. S/he can still be included in an analysis of oedema because any child with oedema is severely malnourished.
- Weight: if the child's information on weight is missing you cannot include her/him in the assessment of wasting. S/he can still be included in an analysis of oedema because any child with oedema is severely malnourished.

B3.3.2 Data out of the required range

In most nutrition surveys we are measuring children aged 6–59 months, or children who are 65–110cm tall. Children outside these ranges should not be included in our results. For example, if a child is measured at 112cm, or is only five months old, s/he should not be included in the analysis (see Appendix S1).

B3.3.3 Extreme weight for height data

As well as excluding children for whom we are missing information or who are out of the required range, we also exclude children who have an extremely high or low WFH during data cleaning. By 'extreme' we mean biologically unlikely. It is very unusual to find any child with a WHZ< –4.00 or a WHZ > +5.00. The chances of finding a child with such a low or high WFH are very, very small. It is more likely that either the weight or the height data was wrongly measured, or recorded, or that the WHZ was wrongly calculated.

If you find a child with a WHZ outside of these limits (less than –4.00 WHZ or more than +5.00 WHZ) you should first check your calculation of WHZ. If the calculation is correct then you must assume that the weight or height figure is wrong. Exclude the child from further analysis.[1]

---

[1] These exclusion criteria are valid if the mean WFH z-score for the survey sample is more than –1.5 z-scores. In very extreme famine conditions, where many children are severely malnourished and the mean WFH z-score for the survey sample is less than –1.5 z-scores, it is possible there may be children with WHZ<–4.00 and the results are not false. In this case, you can change the lower level of exclusion to WHZ<–5.00 and the upper level of exclusion to WHZ < +4.00 (see WHO [1995] for more detail on this point).

Example B3.1
Imagine a female child of 75cm whose real weight is 9.0kg. Her real WHZ would be:

$$WHZ = \frac{9.0 - 9.6}{0.852} = -0.70 \text{ z-scores}$$

But if we mistakenly recorded her weight as 6.0kg then we would think her WHZ was:

$$WHZ = \frac{6.0 - 9.6}{0.852} = -4.22 \text{ z-scores}$$

We would have to exclude this child from the rest of the analysis.

B3.3.4 Mistakes we cannot correct

In general, if we cannot correct data then we delete the record or ignore it during analysis. Of course, it is never possible to be sure that data is completely clean because some errors will not look like mistakes.

Example B3.2
If we recorded the weight of the 75cm child described above as 6.9 kg instead of 9.0kg then her WHZ would be:

$$WHZ = \frac{6.9 - 9.6}{0.852} = -3.2 \text{ z-scores}$$

We would not exclude this child for having an extreme WHZ, so the mistake made will not show up during our data cleaning but the mistake will result in the girl being wrongly classified as malnourished. This is why you have to be very careful when taking and recording measurements. Even a small mistake can make a big difference.

B3.3.5 Checking for measurement bias

Measurement bias occurs when the team has not been adequately trained or supervised (see Part E and Appendix S3) or when measuring equipment is faulty. The best way to avoid measurement bias is to be rigorous in training and supervision and to put in place careful checks on the quality of equipment.

Supervisors should check data collection forms at the end of each day to see if WHZ are feasible and to see if oedema is being realistically reported. There are two other useful methods to check the quality of anthropometric data collected during a nutrition assessment after the data has been collected. The second is best undertaken with a computer.

- Assess the distribution of the final decimal for height and weight. This will tell you if the survey workers are rounding weights and height to the nearest kilogram or centimetre, respectively. You can do this by reviewing the data forms and seeing if there is over-representation of values ending in .0 and .5.
- The standard deviation of the z-scores for WFH and HFA. This tells you if there has been substantial random error injected into the measurements. You would normally expect the standard deviation to be between 0.8 and 1.2 (Michael Golden, personal communication). It is likely to be the lower end of this range if the prevalence of malnutrition is very high. If the standard deviation is outside of this range the quality of the data collection should be further investigated. Calculating the HAZ and their standard deviation can tell you how accurately age was recorded. This may be important for variables which are age-dependent.

If these two data checks give you bad results – if, for example, you find that the teams have been rounding up the height or weight measurements – then you should comment on this in the assessment report. There is little more you can do about this problem for the current assessment; however, you should make sure that the teams do not repeat the mistake in their next survey.

Once you have finished the data cleaning you can start with the analysis.

B3.4 Description of the sample

The first step in an analysis of an anthropometric survey is to describe the sample by producing tables showing the distribution of characteristic variables, such as sex and age.

B3.4.1 Age and sex breakdown of the sample

You should always include an age–sex breakdown of your survey sample to indicate whether the sample is representative of the age group you originally targeted for your survey (usually children aged 6–59 months for anthropometric surveys). For example, a distribution according to age will show whether or not the sample under- or over-represents any particular age group. An under-representation of an age group may reflect higher mortality in that age group, or a bias in the survey (for example, too many young children because the older children were playing outside the house and were not measured). In the same way, a distribution according to sex allows us to verify that both sexes are equally distributed, and that no selection bias has occurred.

A standard table showing the distribution of the age and sex of a sample is shown over the page (Table B3.3). This table should be presented in the results section of every nutrition assessment report to show any sex or age sampling bias. The table is easy to fill in – you simply have to add up how many boys and girls there are in each age group, and put these figures in the first and third columns. Then fill in the cell percentages (see below for explanation).

The age groups proposed here are 6–17 months, 18–29 months, 30–41 months, 42–53 and 54–59 months. The age groups are centred around whole years, because many ages are misreported and age biasing is towards the full years. For example, a child may be said to be one year old but in fact is only ten months old.

Table B3.3 How to fill in the table for distribution of age and sex of sample

	Boys		Girls		Total		Ratio
	No.	%	No.	%	No.	%	Boy:girl
6–17 months							
18–29 months							
30–41 months							
42–53 months							
54–59 months							
Total							

Percentage of boys in this age group = 100 × (boys in age group/total number of children in age group)

Percentage of girls in this age group = 100 × (girls in age group/total number of children in age group)

Percentage of all children in age group = 100 × (children in age group/total number of children)

Ratio of boys to girls in this age group = boys/girls in the selected age group

An example of a form filled in like this is given opposite in Table B3.4.

Table B3.4 Example of a table showing the distribution of age and sex of sample

	Boys		Girls		Total		Ratio
	No.	%	No.	%	No.	%	Boy:girl
6–17 months	96	47.8	105	52.2	201	22.3	1.1
18–29 months	102	48.3	109	51.7	211	23.5	1.1
30–41 months	99	52.1	91	47.9	190	21.1	0.9
42–53 months	96	48.7	101	51.3	197	21.9	1.05
54–59 months	51	51	49	49	100	11.1	1.0
Total	444	49.4	455	50.6	899	100	1.0

Another useful to way to look at the age and sex distribution of the population is to create a population pyramid like the one shown below. The population pyramid should use the same age groups as the table to allow for the biases in age reporting described above. A population pyramid allows you to see the age/sex distribution graphically.

Figure B3.2 Example of a population pyramid for an anthropometric survey

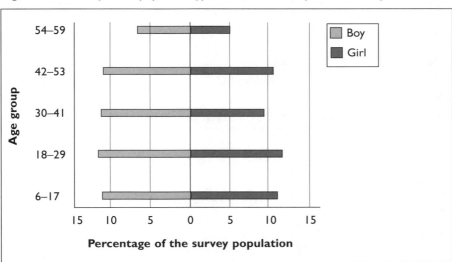

B3.4.2 Checking to see if the sample has any sex or age bias

The ratio of boys to girls allows us to verify that the sample was not biased in terms of sex. As a general rule, if the total ratio is between 0.9 and 1.1 then you can be confident that there was no sex bias in the selection.

Example B3.4
You take a sample of 510 children aged 6–59 months. If you find 256 boys and 254 girls, the sex ratio would be 1.01. This is acceptable: there is no sex bias. However, if you find 306 boys and 204 girls, the sex ratio would be 1.5. This indicates a sex bias in the sampling. You need to investigate why this bias exists and explain it in your report. If the bias is very extreme you may need to re-do the survey.

A normal distribution by age group (for a population aged 6–59 months in the developing world) is shown below in Table B3.5. The distribution of your age groups (like the one in table B3.2 above) should not vary too much from this if the sample is unbiased, ie, the percentage total column should be about the same for all unbiased samples. Note that the 54–59 months age group has a lower percentage than the other groups shown because this group only covers a six-month band and the other groups all cover a 12-month band.

Table B3.5 Typical demographic distribution for children aged 6–59 months in the developing world (WHO, 2000)

	Boys %	Girls %	Total %
6–17 months	12.5	11.4	23.9
18–29 months	13.1	12.4	25.5
30–41 months	11.4	11.0	22.4
42–53 months	10.2	9.0	19.2
54–59 months	5.0	4.0	9.0
Total			100

If you are using a population pyramid, you look at it to see if there is a relatively uniform distribution across the youngest four age-bands with a top age-band about half the size of the others. If the pyramid looks very different from the one shown in Figure B3.2 you need to investigate why.

Reasons for age/sex bias

A comparison of your survey sample's age and sex distribution with either the standard pyramid or standard table shown above may show differences. These differences may be due to one of the following:

- during the survey, one sex (either boys or girls), or age group (older children who are out playing) was less likely to be measured
- either boys or girls or a certain age group suffered higher mortality rates in the past.

The first type of bias is due to a faulty selection procedure and indicates that the survey methodology was not strictly adhered to. This kind of thing can happen if a population believes that a certain age group should not be shown to strangers, or if one sex is hidden. You need to make every effort during your survey to prevent this from happening.

The second type of bias is a real bias in the survey population itself. If you find that there are 'gaps' in the pyramid, or that the percentage of one age group or sex is lower than expected then it may be because this group has suffered excess mortality in the past (see Section D1.3).

If you find either an age or a sex bias in your survey sample you need to investigate why they exist. Is it because of mortality (this involves checking your mortality results) or is it due to a failure in the sampling methods? Age biases in particular can be a serious problem for anthropometric data because younger children are likely to be more malnourished than older children. This means that if you sample too many young children the prevalence of malnutrition is likely to be artificially raised compared with the actual prevalence of malnutrition. For a more detailed discussion of bias in anthropometric data see Chapter D1.

When you have finished describing the sample in terms of age and sex you can start analysing the anthropometric data.

B3.5 Anthropometric data

There are two approaches to analysing and presenting anthropometric results.

- The first approach estimates the prevalence, or proportion, of children whose WFH index falls below a cut-off value. This approach produces an estimate of the prevalence of malnutrition.
- The second approach describes the mean of the whole distribution of children according to index values. This approach produces an estimate of the mean WFH for the population.

In general, although the two approaches are complementary, the first approach is more popular. In particular, if one of the survey's objectives is to quantify the number of children who may benefit from an intensive feeding programme or from supplementary rations based on a cut-off value of the index, then the first approach is more appropriate.

The second approach is useful when you are assessing change in the nutritional status of a population.[2] However, changes in the mean nutritional status of a population are difficult to interpret because we do not know the physiological implications. For this reason it may actually be more useful to compare the prevalence of low WFH, which is physiologically meaningful, rather than mean WFH, when measuring change in the nutritional status of a population.

Current thinking is that it is more important to know the prevalence of malnutrition in a population than the mean nutrition status of the population. This is because it is useful to know how many people are malnourished and need assistance when you are planning your intervention. You should always present the prevalence data in an assessment report; the reporting of mean WFH is useful, but optional.

B3.6 Calculating prevalence of malnutrition and confidence intervals

Several different analyses of the anthropometric data need to be undertaken and presented in order to make the most of the information collected in an anthropometric survey. These will be explained below. However, a brief explanation of how to calculate a prevalence and a confidence interval will be given first.

B3.6.1 Calculating a prevalence

The prevalence, or proportion, of malnutrition is the number of children who are malnourished (see Section B3.2 for the case definitions of malnourished) in relation to the total number of children in the sample. This is calculated by:

$$\text{prevalence malnourished} = \frac{\text{number of malnourished children}}{\text{total number of children measured}} \times 100$$

---

[2] This is because if you compare two means you can use a smaller sample size than if you compare two proportions. This is statistical fact. Because the mean anthropometric status is based on all children in the sample, it can be estimated with greater precision than the prevalence rate, which is based on a smaller number of children. This means that larger samples are needed to demonstrate significant differences between the prevalence of different samples than would be required to show significant differences between means. In practice, we usually calculate sample size based on an estimate of prevalence (see Chapter B2), because the survey objectives are to estimate prevalence. By using the method which compares two means we can detect smaller significant changes in malnutrition than if we use the method to compare two prevalences.

Example B3.5
If a total of 919 children are measured and 155 children are found to be malnourished, the prevalence of malnutrition is:

$$\text{prevalence malnutrition} = \frac{155}{919} \times 100$$

$$= 16.9\%$$

B3.6.2 Confidence intervals

Results should always be presented with their confidence intervals (CI), except for an exhaustive survey which includes all eligible children in the population. Confidence intervals have already been explained in Chapter B2 and Appendix S6.

A CI is a range around an estimate. When we undertake a survey using sampling we calculate a prevalence rate of malnutrition for the sample. This prevalence is only an estimate of the true population prevalence: in order to know the true population prevalence we would have to measure every child. So when we present our sample prevalence we have to also present a range around the value which corresponds to the precision of the estimate. This range, or confidence interval, has a 95% chance of including the true prevalence of malnutrition in the whole population.

The formula to calculate a confidence interval (d) is:

$$d = \pm 1.96\, SE$$

where, SE = standard error of the sample proportion

So,

The upper confidence interval = estimated prevalence + 1.96 * SE
The lower confidence interval = estimated prevalence − 1.96 * SE

In order to calculate a confidence interval, we first have to calculate the standard error. Detailed instructions for how to calculate the standard error and CIs by hand and using Excel for both random and cluster surveys are given in Appendix S7.

Note that the size of the standard error, and hence the size of confidence intervals, will be different depending on the sampling scheme: simple random and systematic sampling will usually produce a lower standard error, all other things being equal, than cluster sampling (see Sections B2.2–B2.5 for more information on this point).

B3.7 Calculation of nutrition indicators

The estimates of global, moderate and severe acute malnutrition, in terms of both z-scores and percentage of the median, should always be presented. All results should include a prevalence and confidence interval.

The definitions of malnutrition are given below (see subsection B1.4.1 for further explanation).

Prevalence expressed in z-scores

Global acute malnutrition prevalence:
Proportion of children with WFH <–2 z-scores and/or oedema

Moderate acute malnutrition prevalence:
Proportion of children with WFH <–2 z-scores and WFH > = –3 z-scores

Severe acute malnutrition prevalence:
Proportion of children with WFH <–3 z-scores and/or oedema

Prevalence expressed in percentage of the median

Global acute malnutrition prevalence:
Proportion of children with WFH < 80% and/or oedema

Moderate acute malnutrition prevalence:
Proportion of children with WFH < 80% and WFH > = 70%

Severe acute malnutrition prevalence:
Proportion of children with WFH < 70% and/or oedema

The steps to calculate the prevalence rates for WHZ are described below.

1. Begin by classifying all data collected according to the WFH reference table and the presence of oedema (already done in the sample form presented in table 3.1)
2. Determine the number of children with oedema = A
3. Determine the number of children with WFH <–3 z-scores but without oedema = B
4. Determine the number of children with WFH <–2 z-scores but without oedema = C
5. Global malnutrition will be C + A

6. Moderate malnutrition will be C – B
7. Severe malnutrition will be B + A
8. Do not count children twice. For example, a child who has oedema and a WFH <–3 z-scores should not be counted as two cases of severe malnutrition.

Then you can calculate the rates of malnutrition.

Example B3.6
We will use the data from the sample anthropometric form (Table B3.1) to illustrate these calculations:

	Number	Calculation for prevalence	Prevalence
Oedema (A)	2		
WFH: < –3 z-scores without oedema (B)	2		
WFH: < –2 z-scores without oedema (C)	6		
Global (A + C) < –2 z-scores or oedema	8	= 100 × (8/30)	26.7%
Moderate (C – B) < –2 z-scores and > –3 z-scores), without oedema	4	= 100 × (4/30)	13.3%
Severe (A + B) < –3 z-scores or oedema	4	= 100 × (4/30)	13.3%

The procedure for WHM is exactly the same:

1. Begin by classifying all data collected according to the WFH reference table and the presence of oedema (already done in the sample form)
2. Determine the number of children with oedema = A
3. Determine the number of children with WFH <70% but without oedema = B
4. Determine the number of children with WFH <80% but without oedema = C
5. Global malnutrition will be C + A
6. Moderate malnutrition will be C – B
7. Severe malnutrition will be B + A
8. Do not count children twice. For example, a child who has oedema and a WHM <70% should not be counted as two cases of severe malnutrition.

Example B3.7
We will use the data from the sample anthropometric form (Table B3.1).

	Number	Calculation for prevalence	Prevalence
Oedema (A)	2		
WFH: <70% median without oedema (B)	1		
WFH: <80% median without oedema (C)	5		
Global (A + C) < 80% or oedema	7	= 100 × (7/30)	23.3%
Moderate (C – B) <80% and > = 70%, without oedema	4	= 100 × (4/30)	13.3%
Severe (A + B) < 70% or oedema	3	= 100 × (3/30)	10.0%

You are now ready to fill in all the anthropometric results tables.

B3.8 Presenting the results of anthropometric data

All reports of emergency nutrition assessments should present the anthropometric results in the tables that are shown and explained below.

B3.8.1 Summary anthropometric results tables

Tables B3.6 and B3.7 summarise the anthropometric results of a survey.[3]

Table B3.6 Prevalence of acute malnutrition based on weight-for-height z-scores and/or oedema

	6–59 months (n = **XX**)
Prevalence of global acute malnutrition (< –2 z-score and/or oedema)	XX % (95% CI XX–XX)
Prevalence of moderate acute malnutrition (< –2 z-score and >= –3 z-scores)	XX % (95% CI XX–XX)
Prevalence of severe acute malnutrition (< –3 z-score and/or oedema)	XX % (95% CI XX–XX)

The prevalence of oedema is XX%

---

[3] You should present the standard error and design effect calculated for the prevalence of global acute malnutrition with table B3.6. This information will allow you to compare statistically the results of the current survey with other surveys (see section D1.1.1). This information can be obtained from CSAMPLE in Epilnfo.

Table B3.7 Prevalence of acute malnutrition based on weight-for-height percentage of the median and/or oedema

	6–59 months (n = **XX**)
Prevalence of global acute malnutrition *(<80% and/or oedema)*	XX % (95% CI XX–XX)
Prevalence of moderate acute malnutrition *(<80% and >= 70%)*	XX % (95% CI XX–XX)
Prevalence of severe acute malnutrition *(<70% and/or oedema)*	XX % (95% CI XX–XX)

The prevalence of oedema is XX%

Example B3.8

To illustrate how to fill in these tables, we will use data from a survey in District A.

Total number of children: 926
Total number of children with oedema: 0
Total number of children with WHZ< −2.00 and no oedema: 180

$$\text{prevalence of global acute malnutrition} = 100 \times \frac{(180 + 0)}{926}$$

$$= 19.4\%$$

$$\text{prevalence of oedema} = 100 \times 0$$

$$= 0\%$$

If we know that the confidence intervals are 15.6–23.2% (see Section S7.1.2, Appendix S7 for this calculation), we can fill in the table.
SE = 1.93 (see calculation in Appendix S8.1.2)
Design effect = 1.7 (taken from CSAMPLE)

Table B3.8 Example of table showing the prevalence of acute malnutrition based on weight-for-height z-scores and/or oedema

	6–59 months (n = 926)
Prevalence of global acute malnutrition *(< −2 z-score and/or oedema)*	(n = 180) 19.4% (95% C.I. 15.6–23.2%)

The prevalence of oedema is 0%.
Standard error for global acute malnutrition = 1.93
Design effect = 1.7

You repeat this process to fill in each of the boxes in Tables B3.6 and B3.7.

B3.8.2 Age-specific prevalence of malnutrition

It is standard practice to report the prevalence of malnutrition by age-specific groups. This is important because the prevalence of malnutrition may be higher in one age group than another.

The table below is the standard one used to report age-specific prevalence of malnutrition defined by low WFH z-scores and/or oedema in nutrition surveys. Children with oedema have their own column. These children should only be included in the oedema column and should not be put into any other column, even if they have low WFH.

The standard age groups are as follows: 6–17 months, 18–29 months, 30–41 months, 42–53 months and 54–59 months. (These age groups are again centred around whole years – 12, 24, 36 months, etc. This is intended to balance the bias towards the reporting of age in whole years.)

Table B3.9 Prevalence of acute malnutrition by age, based on weight-for-height z-scores and oedema

Age (mths)	Total no.	Severe wasting (< –3 z-score) No.	%	Moderate wasting (>= –3 and < –2 z-score) No.	%	Normal (> = –2 z-score) No.	%	Oedema No.	%
6–17									
18–29									
30–41									
42–53									
54–59									
Total									

Percentage of all children < –3 z-scores and in this age group = 100× (number < –3 z-scores/total no. of children in sample)	Percentage of all children > = –3 z-scores < –2 z-scores and in this age group = 100× (number > = –3 and < –2 z-scores/total no. of children in sample)	Percentage of all children > = –2 z-scores and in this age group = 100× (number > = –2 z scores/ total no. of children in sample)	Percentage of all children with oedema in this age group = 100× (number with oedema/total no. of children in sample)

An identical table is used to show the age-specific prevalence of malnutrition defined by low WHM and/or oedema.

Table B3.10 Prevalence of acute malnutrition by age, based on weight-for-height percentage of the median and oedema

		Severe wasting (<70% median)		Moderate wasting (>= 70% <80% median)		Normal (> = 80% median)		Oedema	
Age (mths)	Total no.	No.	%	No.	%	No.	%	No.	%
6–17									
18–29									
30–41									
42–53									
54–59									
Total									

Example B3.9

To practise filling in one of these tables we can use the data from the sample anthropometric data form (Table B3.1). Let us take the youngest age group first. Two children are in this age category (child number '5' and child number '13'). So the total number of children of this age is two. Neither of these children has a WHZ <−3.00, so that column equals zero. Child number '5' has WHZ = −2.19, so he should be entered under the moderate malnutrition column. Child number '13' has a normal WHZ so she is entered under that column. There are no children with oedema in this age group, so that column is zero. Continue this process for each age group. Then fill in the percentage values as explained in Table B3.9. The correct results can be seen in Table B3.11.

Table B3.11 Example of a table showing the prevalence of acute malnutrition by age, based on weight-for-height z-scores and oedema

Age (mths)	Total no.	Severe wasting (< –3 z-score)		Moderate wasting (>= –3 and < –2 z-score)		Normal (> = –2 z-score)		Oedema	
		No.	%	No.	%	No.	%	No.	%
6–17	2	0	0	1	3.3	1	3.3	0	0
18–29	9	2	6.7	1	3.3	6	20.0	0	0
30–41	6	0	0	1	3.3	5	16.7	0	0
42–53	11	0	0	0	0	10	33.3	1	3.3
54–59	2	0	0	1	3.3	0	0	1	3.3
Total	30	2	6.7	4	13.3	22	73.3	2	6.7

For example, $100 \times (2/30) = 6.7$ %.

B3.8.3 Distributions showing the prevalence of malnutrition according to sex

It is standard practice to look at the prevalence of malnutrition according to sex. You need to fill in a table like the one below for this.

Table B3.12 Prevalence of acute malnutrition based on weight-for-height z-scores and/or oedema by sex

	Boys n = XX	Girls n = XX
Prevalence of global acute malnutrition (< –2 z-score and/or oedema)	XX % (95% CI XX–XX)	XX % (95% CI XX–XX)
Prevalence of moderate acute malnutrition (< –2 score and >= –3 z-score)	XX % (95% CI XX–XX)	XX % (95% CI XX–XX)
Prevalence of severe acute malnutrition (< –3 z-score and/or oedema)	XX % (95% CI XX–XX)	XX % (95% CI XX–XX)

The prevalence of oedema is XX%.

B3.8.4 Distributions showing the population according to WFH and oedema

The final anthropometric results table should show the distribution of WFH with respect to the presence of oedema. This allows for the differentiation of children presenting with kwashiorkor from those presenting with marasmic kwashiorkor. It is important to present these results, as children with marasmic kwashiorkor are at greater risk of death than those with either marasmus or kwashiorkor alone.

Table B3.11 Distribution of acute malnutrition and oedema based on weight-for-height z-scores

	< –2 z-score	>= –2 z-score
Oedema present	Marasmic kwashiorkor (n = XX) XX%	Kwashiorkor (n = XX) XX%
Oedema absent	Marasmic (n = XX) XX%	Normal (n = XX) XX%

Example B3.10

To practise filling in one of these tables we can use the data from the sample anthropometric data form (Table B3.1). In the sample, two children have oedema (child number '6' and child number '26'). One of these children has oedema and low WHZ (child 26) and the other has oedema but normal WHZ (child 6). Six children have low WHZ with no oedema and the rest are normal. Thus, the results table should be filled in as below.

Table B3.14 Example of table showing the distribution of acute malnutrition and oedema based on weight-for-height z-scores

	< –2 z-score	>= –2 z-score
Oedema present	Marasmic kwashiorkor (n = 1) 3.3%	Kwashiorkor (n = 1) 3.3%
Oedema absent	Marasmic (n = 6) 20%	Normal (n = 22) 73.3%

B3.9 Presentation of the z-scores distribution and mean

Once you have filled in all the anthropometric tables described above, you have finished the analysis section that produces estimates of the prevalence of malnutrition in the population. This section describes how to produce a mean value for the WFH z-scores and how to plot a graph of the distribution of the z-scores in your survey.

B3.9.1 Plotting WFH distribution curves

The distribution of WFH z-scores can be plotted on a graph and compared with the reference population. Distribution curves of z-scores give a complete picture of the nutrition status of the whole population, which can be compared with that of the reference population.

To calculate a frequency distribution curve, the range of z-scores from < −4.00 to > +5.00[4] is broken down into a number of intervals, and the proportion of children within each interval is calculated. This data is used to plot the frequency distribution curve. This is normally easier to do with a computer programme (like Microsoft Excel) which can draw a graph, than by hand (explained in Save the Children, 2003, on the CD-ROM that accompanies this manual).

In order to plot the data on a graph, you need to create a table like the one below. This table shows us how much of the sample population falls between various ranges of the WHZ measure.

Example B3.11
Table B3.15 shows the frequency distribution of z-scores for children from the District A sample and the distribution for the reference children.

Column 1   shows the range of WHZ. Row −3.75 means the children who are >= −4.00 and < −3.75

Column 2   shows the number of children in the total sample in this range of WHZ

Column 3   shows the proportion of children from the total sample in this range of WHZ (to get this number divide the number of children in a particular range by the total number of children, for example: for the proportion of children in the row −3.75 WHZ [(6/927) × 100] = 0.6)

Column 4   shows the proportion of children in the reference population in this range. This figure does not change − keep the same column for all surveys.

Table B3.15 Frequency distribution of z-scores for the District A survey and the reference population (combined sexes)

1	2	3	4
WHZ range	**Number of children in this range in survey**	**Proportion in survey population**	**Proportion in reference population**
<−4.00	0	0	0
−3.75	6	0.6	0.02

---

[4] Note that this range is the same as the permissible upper and lower limits of the WFH z-score that you use for cleaning the anthropometric data (see subsection B3.3.3). This means that all the children will be included on the graph.

1	2	3	4
WHZ range	Number of children in this range in survey	Proportion in survey population	Proportion in reference population
−3.25	11	1.2	0.1
−2.75	39	4.2	0.45
−2.25	124	13.4	1.59
−1.75	199	21.5	4.31
−1.25	247	26.6	9.13
−0.75	169	18.2	15.06
−0.25	79	8.5	19.33
0.25	43	4.6	19.33
0.75	8	0.9	15.06
1.25	1	0.1	9.13
1.75	1	0.1	4.31
2.25	0	0	1.59
2.75	0	0	0.45
3.25	0	0	0.1
3.75	0	0	0.02
4.25	0	0	0
4.75	0	0	0
>5.00	0	0	0
	927	**100**	**100**

Then use this data to make a graph like in the one Figure B3.3.

B3.9.2 Population mean WFH z-score measurements

The mean WHZ is sometimes used to describe a population's nutrition status. This is calculated as:

$$\text{mean WHZ} = \frac{\text{sum of all WFH z-scores}}{\text{number of children measured}}$$

In some situations it may be useful to calculate the mean WHZ in order to compare current survey results with older survey results. Section S7.2 in Appendix S7 describes how to calculate confidence intervals for the population mean WFH z-score. However, comparison of the two means gathered from cluster sample surveys requires more complex statistical formulae than are currently readily available in EpiInfo.

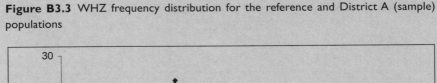

Figure B3.3 WHZ frequency distribution for the reference and District A (sample) populations

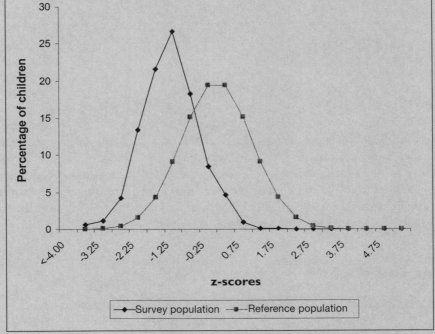

From this type of graph you can compare the distribution of z-scores in your sample population with the reference population.

In Figure B3.3 we can see that the sample population's WHZ distribution has shifted to the left compared with the reference population. This indicates that the population in District A are malnourished compared with the reference population.

B3.10 Vaccination data

Information about how to collect vaccination data is presented in subsection A4.5.4. The analysis of these results is presented here because it is similar to that for anthropometric data.

The estimated prevalence of vaccination should be calculated and presented in a similar way to prevalence of acute malnutrition. Tables should look like the one below:

Table B3.16 Vaccination coverage: BCG for 6–59 months and measles for 9–59 months

	BCG n = XX	Measles (with card) n = XX	Measles (with card or confirmation from mother) n = XX
YES	(n=XX) XX % (95% CI XX–XX)	(n=XX) XX % (95% CI XX–XX)	(n=XX) XX % (95% CI XX–XX)

You should calculate the prevalence and confidence intervals of vaccination in exactly the same way as you do for acute malnutrition (explained in Section B3.6). The analysis of the measles vaccination should only include children aged nine months and over because measles vaccines are not generally given to children less than nine months of age. However, if an objective of the survey is the evaluation of coverage achieved by a recent emergency mass measles vaccination campaign which targeted children aged six months and over, then the questionnaire and the analysis should include all the children aged 6–59 months. An example of a completed table for vaccination results is given below.

Table B3.17 Example of a table showing vaccination coverage: BCG for 6–59 months and measles for 9–59 months

	BCG n = 905	Measles (with card) n = 886	Measles (with card or confirmation from mother) n = 886
YES	(n = 189) 20.9% (95% CI 13.1–8.7%)	(n = 37) 4.2% (95% CI 0.9–7.4%)	(n = 272) 30.7% (95% CI 19.2–42.2%)

B3.11 Morbidity data

As described in subsection A4.5.2 the best way to get information on a population is usually from MoH staff and through discussions with women or community leaders. This type of information should be presented in the text of your assessment report.

In some surveys, morbidity data is collected during the anthropometric survey from children's carers. If you decide to do this then you must use standardised case definitions which are explained to each survey respondent. Without such standardisation each respondent will report something different and, at the end, you cannot calculate a period prevalence of anything. Moreover, without case standardisation different surveys cannot be compared and those who analyse the data cannot tell if the period prevalence is low or high for a particular population.

In general, morbidity data collected in the anthropometric questionnaires is presented in frequency tables showing simple proportions. Table B3.18 should be presented first. This shows the total number of children reporting any illness.

Table B3.18 Prevalence of reported illness in children in the two weeks prior to interview (n =)

	6–59 months
Prevalence of reported illness	XX % (95% CI XX–XX)

Then create a table showing what illnesses were reported.

Table B3.19 Symptom breakdown in the children in the two weeks prior to interview (n =)

	6–59 months
Diarrhoea	XX % (95% CI XX–XX)
Cough/breathing difficulties	XX % (95% CI XX–XX)
Fever	XX % (95% CI XX–XX)
Measles	XX % (95% CI XX–XX)
Other	XX % (95% CI XX–XX)

Example B3.12
You can practise filling in morbidity tables using the data from the sample anthropometric form in Section B3.2.

Total children =	30
Total with diarrhoea =	4
Total with cough =	2
Total with fever =	2
Total with measles =	0
Total with other =	3

So total ill =   4 + 2 + 2 + 3   = 11

Prevalence of illness = $\dfrac{11}{30} \times 100$

=   36.7%

Therefore your results should look like Table B3.20.

Table B3.20 Example of table showing prevalence of reported illness in children in the two weeks prior to interview (n = 30)

	6–59 months
Prevalence of reported illness	36.7%

To calculate the symptom breakdown among children who reported illness:

Total ill children =   30
Total with diarrhoea =   4

Proportion with diarrhoea = $\frac{4}{30} \times 100$

=   13.3%

Therefore your results should look like Table B3.21.

Table B3.21 Symptom breakdown in the children who reported illness in the two weeks prior to interview (n = 30)

	6–59 months
Diarrhoea	13.3%
Cough	6.7%
Fever	6.7%
Measles	0%
Other	10%

The interpretation of morbidity data collected in an anthropometric questionnaire is not straightforward. This is discussed further in subsection A5.2.1.

Summary

- Anthropometric data should always be prepared and cleaned prior to analysis. This means excluding children who have extreme anthropometric data.
- A standard set of anthropometric results tables must be filled in for every

nutrition survey. This allows agencies to compare the results of different surveys. The standard tables include:

- sample distribution of age and sex
- summary anthropometric results tables (for WHM and WHZ)
- age-specific prevalence of malnutrition (for WHM and WHZ)
- sex-specific prevalence of malnutrition (for WHM and WHZ)
- distributions according to WFH and oedema.

• Vaccination and morbidity data should also be presented in a standard format.

Part C
Assessing the rate of mortality

In this part of the manual we discuss the importance of obtaining information on the mortality rates of the population which you are surveying in an emergency nutrition assessment. Malnutrition and mortality are inextricably linked and a joint analysis of both of these factors helps you to understand the situation better and therefore make more appropriate recommendations for interventions.

This section follows the pattern of previous sections: theory, data collection methods and analysis. The first chapter discusses the association between malnutrition and mortality and common measures of mortality employed in emergencies. The second chapter describes how to collect mortality data. The final chapter explains how to analyse mortality data. The joint interpretation of mortality, anthropometric and malnutrition causes data is described in Chapter D1.

Chapter C1
Key concepts

This chapter describes the importance of collecting mortality data in emergencies. The relationship between malnutrition and mortality is discussed. Some definitions of the most commonly used measures of mortality in emergencies are given.

C1.1 The relationship between malnutrition and mortality

The Unicef conceptual framework of the causes of malnutrition (Figure A1.1) shows both mortality and malnutrition at the top of the model. Mortality is the ultimate outcome of health and nutrition conditions and provides an overall picture of a population's health status. While the causes of mortality go beyond those related to malnutrition, there is evidence to show that malnutrition is among the principal causes of mortality in emergencies.

Figure C1.1 Wasting and mortality in refugee and displaced populations in Africa (Source: ACC/SCN, 1994)

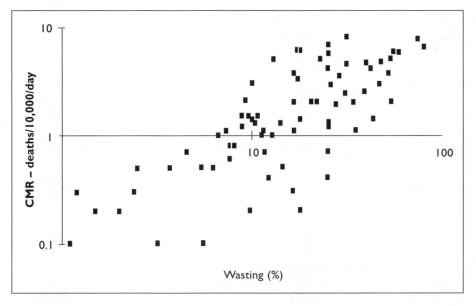

Figure C1.1 shows the association between wasting and mortality across emergency-affected African populations. You can see that the relationship between the two is quite strong but not constant. This means it is not possible to predict the mortality rate on the basis of prevalence of malnutrition, or vice versa. The reason for this is that risk of infection changes in different contexts and mortality is linked to the risk of infection. Hence, the mortality rate associated with a given level of acute malnutrition changes in different contexts.

When malnutrition becomes widespread in a population, mortality rates increase rapidly. When multiple causes of malnutrition exist they appear to interact with one another, resulting in a greater combined impact on malnutrition and mortality than would be expected if the causes were acting in isolation (Young, 2004).

Problems of defining the term 'famine'

The fact that malnutrition and mortality do not always increase in tandem has led to difficulties in defining what exactly a famine is. There is no standard, universally accepted definition of famine.

Current views of famine have evolved from the historical definition that was based only on lack of food and the presence of widespread hunger and starvation. Famine is now more usually characterised by excess mortality and high malnutrition in all age groups of the population. Moreover, famine is now viewed as a process, gradually worsening until finally resulting in a considerable number of excess deaths. The exact level of mortality and/or prevalence of malnutrition which can be declared a 'famine', however, cannot be given. Chapter D1 discusses cut-offs for determining the severity of a mortality rate and malnutrition prevalence.

C1.2 Common measures of mortality in emergencies

In emergency situations mortality is normally reported in two ways: crude mortality rate (CMR) and under-five mortality rate (U5MR). These rates are defined as:

- **CMR:** the rate of death in the entire population, including both sexes and all ages
- **U5MR:** the rate of death among children below five years of age in the population.

In emergency situations, the most commonly used standard population denominator and time period is per 10,000 population per day. However, both CMR and U5MR can be expressed with different standard population denominators and for different time periods – eg, deaths per 1,000 population per month.

The definitions for calculating the CMR and U5MR are in the box below.

> **Mortality rates commonly measured in emergencies**
>
> CMR = total deaths/10,000 people/day
>
> U5MR = deaths in children under five/
> 10,000 children under five/day

Demographers use many other measures of mortality including age-specific death rates.[1] It is beyond the scope of this manual to describe all the methods. We will focus on the most commonly used measures of mortality in emergencies: the CMR and U5MR. You need to be careful when comparing the rates of mortality calculated in this way with those from other sources.

C1.3 Use of mortality data in emergencies
C1.3.1 CMR data

The CMR is the most important public health indicator for all populations, particularly for societies in crisis. It is essential that humanitarian organisations have some understanding of the CMR in emergencies.

In particular, the CMR is useful for (SMART, 2003):

- assessing the overall severity of the situation for a population under stress
- informing and prioritising resource allocation between emergencies
- advocating the urgency of an intervention
- triangulating other information about the emergency situation
- calibrating surveillance data[2]

---

[1] For example, Unicef defines its infant mortality rate (in the 'State of the World's Children') as: 'the probability of dying between birth and exactly one year of age expressed per 1,000 live births'. The Unicef under-five mortality rate is 'the probability of dying between birth and exactly five years of age expressed per 1,000 live births'. Note that this is entirely different from the calculation of an age-specific mortality rate of children under five years divided by the number of children in this age group. The Unicef 'rate' will be much higher than the age-specific rate because it counts all the deaths over the five years, whereas the age-specific rate counts only one year's deaths.

[2] Routine surveillance data from clinics may systematically over- or under-estimate the mortality rate in a population. If you undertake a cross-sectional retrospective mortality survey then you may be able to estimate the extent of the bias in the clinic reporting. Then you may be able to re-calibrate the data from the clinics. The extent to which calibration is possible depends on the extent to which the data is representative and how this has changed over time.

- documenting the crisis and assessing the overall impact of humanitarian interventions.[3]

C1.3.2 U5MR data

As with under-five malnutrition, under-five mortality rates are likely to be a useful indicator of the situation in the whole population, as mortality rates in this age group are likely to be most sensitive to shocks. Furthermore, U5MR provide useful information about the situation of young children. Unlike malnutrition, however, under-five mortality rates are not always reported, and crude mortality rates are often preferred. This is because most organisations collect CMR data and use the same sample size to estimate U5MR in emergency situations. This usually means that the U5MR is much less precise than the CMR – often too low to be of value for decision-making.

It should be noted that U5MR is not an appropriate indicator for initial assessments undertaken where considerable under-five mortality has occurred prior to the start of the follow-up period (eg, initial assessments undertaken very late in an ongoing nutritional emergency) or in situations where mortality is likely to be highest in the adult or elderly population.

C1.4 When to undertake a mortality survey?

Chapter C2 discusses some of the limitations of mortality surveys. A surveillance system for monitoring mortality (eg, by registering deaths or graves, or by providing shrouds) is preferable to a mortality survey and every effort should be made to set up such a system as soon as possible in an emergency. This is because a mortality survey only tells you about past rather than current mortality. Surveys do not tell you if the situation is improving or deteriorating and they can often be biased.

A mortality survey takes time and money and so there is no point in undertaking such a survey unless you need the information and no other agency has reliable and up-to-date mortality information on the population in which you are interested. However, the mortality rate provides useful additional information to help interpret the prevalence and causes of malnutrition and can considerably strengthen the conclusions of an emergency nutrition assessment. Remember, as for nutrition data, you must always be prepared to respond to the findings of a mortality survey, or else you should not collect the information in the first place.

---

[3] This should be done using trend analysis, rather than fixed thresholds. Typically, many organisations provide the package of interventions essential to meet critical needs in emergencies, and hence a change in CMR or U5MR is usually not appropriate for evaluating individual interventions or performance of individual agencies.

Summary

- The mortality rate is the most important public health indicator in all populations, particularly in emergencies.
- The relationship between mortality and malnutrition will vary according to the underlying morbidity pattern and causes of malnutrition.
- The CMR (crude mortality rate) and U5MR (under-five mortality rate) are the two most commonly used mortality rates in emergency assessments:
  - CMR is defined as total deaths/10,000 population/day.
  - U5MR is defined as total under-five deaths/10,000 population of under-fives/day.
- Setting up mortality surveillance systems should be a priority in emergencies. Mortality surveys have many limitations and use up resources. Mortality surveys should only be undertaken if no recent and reliable mortality data are available.

Chapter C2
Measuring mortality

This chapter begins by outlining some general principles about the collection of mortality data. Later sections of the chapter describe how to calculate sample sizes for a cross-sectional retrospective mortality survey. Different questionnaire and recall methods to collect mortality data are outlined. The chapter finishes with a discussion about potential difficulties in collecting mortality data and suggests ways to overcome the difficulties.

C2.1 General principles for measuring mortality in a retrospective cross-sectional survey

Mortality surveillance systems are the recommended method for obtaining an estimate of mortality during an emergency (The Sphere Project, 2004 and Médecins Sans Frontières, 1997). Surveillance requires the ongoing measurement of mortality over time rather than in a one-off survey. Often systems for counting deaths can be put in place fairly quickly, although in situations where the population numbers are rapidly changing due to in- and out-migration the information may be difficult to interpret. The following are common sources of mortality data:

- **Surveillance data:** consult lists if deaths are registered by the local authorities, clinics or hospitals. Surveillance data can often be biased against the most vulnerable. Those who cannot access health services, for example, may not be included in the system.
- **Grave counting**: by counting the number of graves, although this is not always feasible (eg, it is impossible in a setting where bodies are incinerated). This method cannot be used to assess mortality rates prior to displaced people moving, but may be useful in a camp for displaced people if everyone is buried in the same place.
- **Religious authority data**: religious authorities or funeral associations that are responsible for burials, etc, often keep records (in order to keep accounts).

In the absence of such a system or when these systems are known to be very inaccurate, a cross-sectional retrospective mortality survey can be conducted to fill an information gap before the surveillance system can be developed or improved.

There are important differences between anthropometric and mortality surveys. When you estimate the amount of malnutrition in an emergency-affected population the anthropometric data provide a static picture of the present nutritional situation – ie, they provide a cross-sectional, point prevalence estimate at the date of the survey. Mortality data are different. You need to count the number of deaths over a time period (which is past) and obtain a rate. The other big difference between an anthropometric survey and a mortality survey is that a mortality survey gives you information about the average mortality over the recall period but *not* the rate of mortality on the day of the survey. Anthropometric surveys tell you the prevalence of malnutrition on the day of the survey.

Figure C2.1 shows the general principles of a cross-sectional retrospective mortality survey.

Figure C2.1 The general principles of a cross-sectional retrospective mortality survey (Source: Woodruff, 2002)

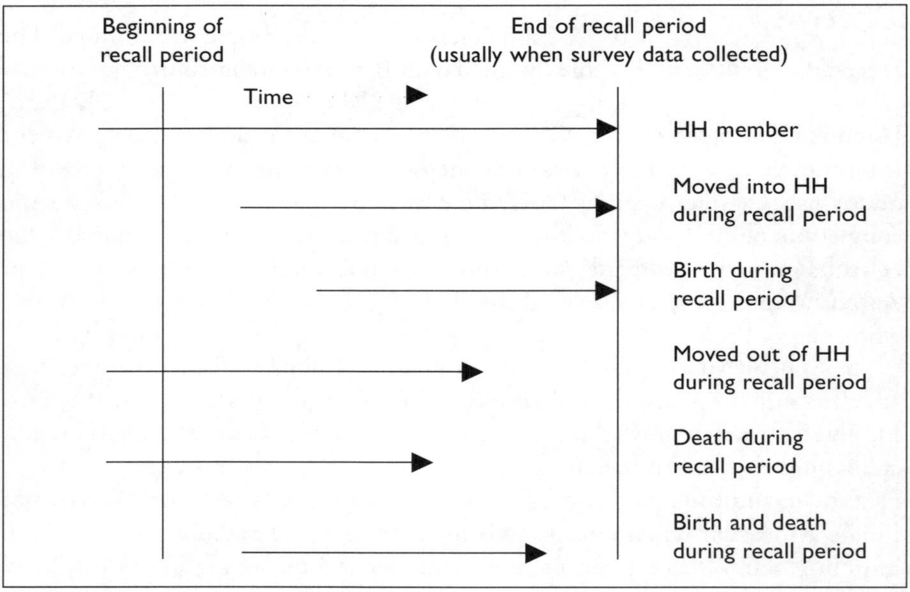

HH = Household

Using Figure C2.1 as a starting point, it is possible to describe key aspects of retrospective mortality surveys (note that some of these topics will be discussed in more detail later in the chapter):

Denominators of mortality rates

The denominator of a mortality rate is the survey sample itself and does not depend on estimates of the population size. The denominator is usually calculated as person-days-at-risk (PDAR). The PDAR is equal to the number of people in the sample multiplied by the number of days covered by the recall period. Person days at risk can be all-age persons (as required for crude mortality rate – CMR) or only under-fives (as required for under-five mortality rate – U5MR).

Recall period

The recall period should be short enough to allow accurate recall of deaths and births, but long enough for the results to detect enough PDAR for statistical precision. Shorter recall periods are preferable in emergencies so that recent mortality rates can be measured – ideally rates which have occurred since the emergency. Longer recall periods require a smaller sample and therefore surveys with longer recall period are faster and cheaper to conduct.

The beginning of the recall period should be a well-known date that everyone in the population can remember, eg, a major holiday or festival (Christmas, beginning of Ramadan, etc) or the day of a ceasefire. In places where accurate records of births and deaths are kept, the date set for the beginning of the recall period can be arbitrarily chosen and determined by the sample size required. The end of the recall period is usually the day of the survey data collection.

Births and deaths

In a mortality survey, living household members report information on births and deaths over the recall period. The recall and reporting of deaths needs to be as complete as possible. A birth should be defined as a live birth. A distinction should be made between live births and stillbirths or miscarriages. Live-born children are defined as those born alive even if the child died immediately after birth. A baby who cried or breathed – if only for a few minutes – is counted as a live birth.

In- and out-migration from the household

Ideally, information about in- and out-migration from the household should be collected during a retrospective mortality survey. However, most agencies do not collect this information during an emergency assessment as it may be relatively time-consuming to do so and usually makes little difference to the calculation of mortality rates.[1] If you decide to exclude in- and out-migration it should be excluded from the denominator and the numerator in the data collection. Therefore the death of someone who migrated into the household within the recall period should be excluded.

---

[1] An exception to this rule may be when a relatively high proportion of the population left their households during the recall period to look for work elsewhere or to join the military. If the mortality rates in the place where they have gone to work are very different from the mortality rates in the survey area then the rates of mortality will be affected.

C2.2 Sampling for a retrospective mortality survey

The principles of sampling for mortality data are similar to those for anthropometric surveys: ie, if you are *not* going to undertake an exhaustive mortality survey of all the households in an area then you need to make sure the households you sample are representative of the whole population (see Chapter B2 for more details on this).

As with an anthropometric survey, you can use simple random, cluster or systematic sampling to collect mortality data. The choice of method to use will depend on a variety of factors including population size, distribution and the amount of information you have about the population.

Anthropometric surveys and mortality surveys are usually carried out at the same time (it would be very rare to only conduct a mortality survey). However, the two types of survey require that you sample different households – the mortality survey requires a sample of all households whereas the anthropometric survey requires a sample of households with children aged 6–59 months. This means that your method for sampling households can be the same – eg, systematic or two-stage cluster sampling – but decisions about which households are eligible for inclusion in the survey are different.

It is important to calculate the sample size required for a mortality survey separately from the sample size calculation required for an anthropometric survey. This is because the two sample sizes may differ according to the rates of mortality or prevalence of malnutrition that you expect to find, the level of precision you are prepared to accept and the design effect you decide to use. There is no point in over-sampling for a mortality survey because surveys take time and can waste resources.

Note that many organisations simply use the same sample size (although not the same households) for mortality assessments as they do for nutrition assessments. For example, if they are undertaking a 30 x 30 cluster anthropometric survey they will also ask about mortality in 30 households in each of 30 clusters. Although this may be a convenient approach it is not strictly correct for the reasons given above (also see Chapter B2).

C2.2.1 Sample size for a mortality survey

As with anthropometric surveys, you need to estimate the rate of mortality you expect in advance of the mortality survey and decide the level of precision you will accept in your survey findings. Higher levels of precision are required when the mortality rate is not expected to be very different from pre-emergency rates, whereas lower levels of precision are acceptable if mortality rates are expected to be excessively high.

The sample size required to measure CMR may be different from the sample size required to measure U5MR. The denominator you will need to estimate

CMR is the PDAR for the whole population (all ages) and the denominator you will need to estimate the U5MR is the PDAR for children under five.

The relative rates of the CMR and U5MR will determine when you need a bigger sample size for each. If both the CMR and the U5MR are relatively low then you will need to visit more households if you are trying to estimate the U5MR as opposed to CMR. This is because there will be fewer PDAR in a household than if you were sampling the whole population.

As with an anthropometric survey, an estimation of design effect is required for the calculation of sample size. The design effect which should be used for a mortality survey may be quite different from that for an anthropometric survey and will depend on the health environment and whether mortality has occurred in specific locations due to conflict. If epidemics and massacres have occurred, making it likely that some clusters in your survey will have extremely high rates of mortality and others very low rates and you will need to use a high design effect (ie, more than 2). As with an anthropometric survey, if simple random sampling is conducted the design effect is 1.

C2.2.2 Software for sample size calculations for a mortality rate

A piece of software for calculating sample sizes for a mortality rate using a cross-sectional retrospective survey has recently been produced. The software (called samplerate) is available on the CD-ROM attached to this manual.[2]

When the programme opens you see like the screen below. The programme is very easy to use – you simply type in the expected rate (for either CMR or U5MR), the error you will accept and the design effect you expect. The Help file describes in detail how to use the software. The number of PDAR you will need is then calculated automatically.

Example C2.1
You expect that the CMR will be 2/10,000/day and you will accept an error of 1/10,000 day. You are using a two-stage cluster design sampling method. You don't expect mortality to be clustered in the population so you use a design effect of 2. Simply adjust the screen using the arrow keys to get the figures you want. The screen will look like the one below.

---

[2] The software can also be downloaded from: http://www.myatt.demon.co.uk/samplexs.htm

```
Sample Size Calculator - Single Rate                      [X]

        Rate :  [2    ▲▼]   per  [10000    ▼]   per  [day    ▼]

      ± Error :  [1    ▲▼]   per 10000 per day

  Design Effect :  [2.0   ▲▼]

            N :  [153664        ]   person-days        [ Help ]
```

In this case you need 153,664 PDAR for your mortality survey. In order to obtain the number of people to be included in the survey the PDAR should be divided by the number of days in the recall period. If the recall period was 90 days 153,664 would be divided by 90 resulting in a sample size of 1,707 people.

C2.2.3 Calculating sample sizes by hand for a mortality rate

You will normally use the samplerate software to calculate sample sizes for a mortality survey. However, if for some reason you do not have access to the software you can use the equations below to calculate the sample size.

Sample sizes for a mortality survey can be calculated using the following formula:

$$n = \frac{\mu}{(\varepsilon \div t)^2} \times k$$

Where:

n = number of person days at risk (PDAR)
μ = rate (eg, 2/10,000 = 0.0002)
t = linked to the confidence interval required:
    90% CI   t = 1.62
    95% CI   t = 1.96
    99% CI   t = 2.57
ε = precision (eg, 1/10,000 = 0.0001)
k = design effect

Example C2.2
The sample size required to estimate a CMR of 2 / 10,000 persons / day with a 95% confidence interval of ± 1 / 10,000 persons / day using *simple random sampling* is:

$$n = \frac{0.0002}{(0.0001/1.96)^2} \times 1$$

= 76,923 PDAR

Number of people required in the sample = $\dfrac{\text{PDAR}}{\text{length of follow-up period in days}}$

For example, with a follow-up period of 90 days:

Number of people = $\dfrac{76,923}{90}$

= 855 people

Example C2.3
Using the same information as in the example above: the sample size required to estimate an U5MR of 4 / 10,000 persons / day with a 95% confidence interval of ± 1 / 10,000 children under five / day in a resident population where there has been a measles outbreak using cluster sampling is:

$$n = \frac{0.0004}{(0.0001/1.96)^2} \times 5$$

= 769,230

If the recall period is 90 days then children required in the sample

= $\dfrac{769,230}{90}$

= 8,547 children are required

C2.2.4 How many households should you visit?

In a survey measuring CMR, the number of people required can be calculated by dividing the sample size by the average number of people per household. In measuring the U5MR, the number of children under five required for the sample can be calculated by dividing by the average number of under-fives per household. It should be noted that the same households are visited for measuring CMR and U5MR. After calculating the sample sizes required for estimating CMR and U5MR, the highest number should be taken as the sample size for the mortality survey.

Example C2.4: number of households required for CMR for a random survey

If your sample size calculations require you to have a sample size of 854 people and the average number of people per household was 5.1 then you would need to assess mortality in 168 households:

Number of households you need to visit = $\dfrac{\text{total number of people required}}{\text{average number of people per household}}$

$= \dfrac{854}{5.1}$

= 167.4 households (this number should be rounded up)

= 168 households

Example C2.5: number of households required for U5MR for a random survey

If your sample size calculations require you to have a sample size of 854 children under five and the average number of children under five per household was 1.7, then you would need to assess mortality in 503 households:

Number of households you need to visit = $\dfrac{\text{total number of children under 5 required}}{\text{average number of children under 5 per household}}$

$= \dfrac{854}{1.7}$

= 502.3 households (this number
should be rounded up)

= 503 households

C2.2.5 Selection of households for a mortality survey

The process of selecting households for a mortality survey is similar to that for anthropometric surveys and depends on which type of sampling you have chosen (simple random, systematic or cluster). However, *all* households, including those with no children aged 6–59 months, must be eligible for selection in a mortality survey. Thus, when you are using two-stage cluster sampling, after the selection of the first household (see Chapter B2) a mortality survey should visit all the subsequent houses to the left or right, including those with no children.

If a mortality survey only includes households with children under the age of five years, a major bias will be introduced. For example, a household without a young child because the last-born child died recently would be excluded and would result in an underestimation of the mortality rate. So we should include this household in the mortality survey for estimating both U5MR and CMR.

C2.3 How long should the recall period be?

The recall period is an important determinant of the survey sample size because the PDAR calculation depends on the number of people at risk (of death) for a given number of days. If you make the recall period longer then you can have a smaller sample of households which usually makes the survey quicker to conduct.

There is no 'correct' length of time for a recall period for retrospective mortality surveys. The recall period you need should, as stated above in Section C2.1, be decided by taking into account the following factors:

- Accuracy: the recall period should be short enough to allow accurate recall.
- Statistical precision: the recall period should be long enough for the results to be meaningful and to have enough PDAR for statistical precision.
- Recent changes in mortality rates: if mortality rates are changing rapidly you may not be interested in the average rate over the last year but rather the average rate over the last few months.
- The population should have a relatively constant mortality rate during the recall period. This may have to be assumed if the information is not available.
- The beginning of the recall period should be a well-known date that everyone in the population remembers – eg, a major holiday or festival (Christmas, beginning of Ramadan, etc) or a political election.

- Seasonality in mortality: if you are trying to measure the impacts on mortality of factors which are not determined by season then your recall period should be chosen to cover several seasons so these effects can be smoothed out.
- Longer recall periods reduce the sample size and therefore speed up the survey.

Balancing out these different factors will mean that you take a different recall period for different surveys.

Example C2.5

You need to assess mortality in a rural population because you have heard that next year's harvest is going to be a failure. The seasonal calendar of events which directly impact on mortality is shown below. The population faces seasonal shortages of food from May to October, but particularly from August to October. Malaria outbreaks occur mainly in January and February. The harvest is normally due in November.

	Jan	Feb	Mar	Apr	May	Jun	Jul	Aug	Sep	Oct	Nov	Dec
Food shortage					X	X	X	XX	XX	XX		
Malaria outbreak	X	X										

Imagine you undertake the mortality assessment in October:

- If you use a recall period of three months you will obtain mortality data which are affected by the worst of the food shortage period.
- If you use a recall period of six months you will obtain mortality data which are affected by the moderate food shortage as well as the more severe food shortage.

Other things being equal, your estimate of the CMR using the shorter recall period will probably give a higher CMR than the estimate using the longer recall period.

The same would be true if you were estimating the mortality for the malaria season in a mortality assessment in March. If you took too long a recall period then you would dilute the effect of malaria on mortality rates.

In general, most emergency assessments of mortality use a recall period of about 90 days (3 months). In a severe and new crisis it may be more appropriate to use a recall period of 30 days.

C2.4 Three different recall / questionnaire methods for measuring mortality in a retrospective survey in an emergency

At least three different questionnaire methods for measuring mortality are currently used in emergency assessments:

- current household census
- past household census
- previous birth history (PBH).

All the methods available for retrospective mortality surveys need to be tested in a variety of contexts to determine which ones are most suited to which contexts. In the absence of this information no specific method is recommended here.[3]

Note that you calculate the sample size in the same way for all the three questionnaire methods.

C2.4.1 Current household census method

This method, which is probably the most commonly employed, obtains the following information:

- the age (under five and all ages) of each person who lives in the household on the day of the survey
- number of births and deaths (under five and all ages) within household during recall period.

An example of the questionnaire you would fill in for this method of mortality recall is given in Section S6.2, Appendix S6. If household in- and out-migration was expected to be high during the recall period the questionnaire would need to be modified in order to measure this. An explanation of how to calculate mortality rates for this method is given in Chapter C3.

C2.3.2 Past household census method

This method obtains the following information:

- the age (under five and all ages) of each person who lived in the household at beginning of recall period

---

[3] Operational research is being conducted by agencies connected to the SMART initiative to determine the most suitable method for measuring mortality in retrospective surveys in emergencies.

- number of births during recall period
- current status of these individuals separately (all ages and under-fives).

An example of the questionnaire you would fill in for this method of mortality recall is given in Section S6, Appendix S6. If household in- and out-migration was expected to be high during the recall period the questionnaire would need to be modified in order to measure this. An explanation of how to calculate mortality rates for this method is given in Chapter C3.

The principal difference between the past and current household census methods is that the past census conducts a census at the beginning of the recall period and the current census conducts a census at the end of the recall period.

C2.4.3 Previous birth history[4]

This method obtains the following information from women:

- births to women in household in previous five years
- current status for each child born in previous five years.

Figure C2.2 Previous birth history (PBH) method

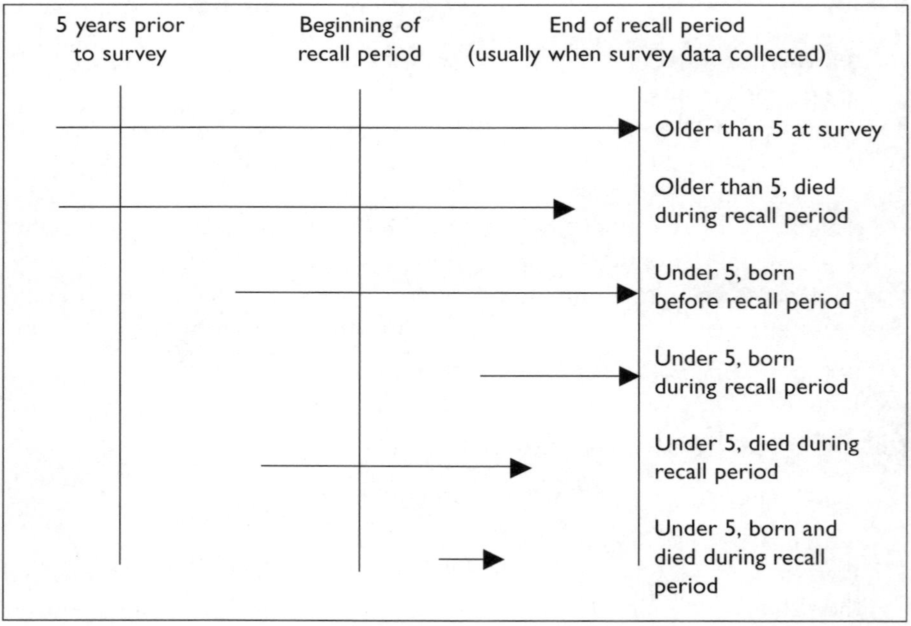

---

[4] The method is described in detail in Myatt et al (2002). The article is on the CD-ROM attached to this manual.

You will notice that this method differs from the previous method because you do not conduct household census and you only collect data on children under five years; therefore, you cannot calculate the CMR. Figure C2.2 outlines the principle of this method. This methodology yields three variables per mother. These are:

- the number of **children at risk**
- the number of **new births** in the survey period
- the number of **new deaths** in the survey period.

An example of the questionnaire you would fill in for this method of mortality recall is given in Section S6.4, Appendix S6. An explanation of how to calculate mortality rates for this method is given in Chapter C3.

C2.5 Difficulties with measuring mortality

As stated above, the most reliable method to collect mortality data is through a surveillance system. The reason for this is that there are problems collecting mortality data through retrospective surveys, including the following.

- **Manipulation of information**: Any emergency assessment is prone to manipulation by a population that has a lot of knowledge and experience of aid programmes. Such manipulation may lead to an overestimation of incidence. The PBH and past census methods may to some extent avoid this problem.
- **Taboo**: In some cultures death is a taboo subject. This makes asking questions about deaths problematic and will lead to an underestimation of mortality.
- **Poor recall of deaths**: Sometimes a traumatised population may not remember all the deaths in the household, especially those of young children. If families have been split up because of insecurity it is possible that they do not know whether someone is alive or dead.
- **Poor recall of live births**: If a child has died very shortly after birth it is possible the family will not remember or will not consider it a live birth. Alternatively, if a live birth is not properly defined by the survey workers then stillbirths may be included in the calculations, resulting in a higher mortality rate (see Section C2.1 for definitions).
- **Determining age**: In many populations people do not know exactly how old they are. As a result, older children may be included in the numerator or denominator of the U5MR calculation which could lead to an overestimation of the rate. This can be overcome by using a detailed local calendar (see Section S2.2, Appendix S2).

- **Recall of date of birth or death:** Many populations are not aware of the exact date, thus it is difficult for them to recall exact dates of birth or death. Again, this problem can be overcome to a certain extent by using a detailed local calendar.
- **Deaths of women or entire household:** If a whole household has died then it is not possible to get information on mortality using any of the methods described above. In the PBH method, *maternal orphans* are excluded by the requirement that only living mothers are interviewed. It might be expected that the survival probabilities of maternal orphans are considerably lower than children whose mothers are still alive. This means that any method based on the PBH question will result in an underestimation of mortality. The degree to which this underestimates mortality will depend upon the maternal mortality rate. Underestimation may be a particular problem in situations of exceptionally high maternal mortality coupled with high under-five mortality due to, for example, HIV/AIDS or malaria epidemic.
- **Time required:** Some of the methods (particularly the past census method), may take a long time at each household.
- **Overestimating mortality:** The past census method may slightly overestimate mortality. This is because we count as under-five deaths those children who were under five at the start of the recall period and would be over five at the end, but who die during the recall period. These children do not contribute to the denominator as they are under five at the start, leading to an overestimation.

C2.6 Causes of death

Information on the cause of death is useful because it can help you to prioritise interventions (see Chapter D1). However, this type of information is often difficult to collect when death takes place outside health facilities. Information collected from family members is generally not very reliable. The best place to get information on the most common causes of death is Ministry of Health (MoH) staff or community leaders. Often religious authorities will also know of an epidemic (see section C2.1).

The problems for collecting data on cause of death from household surveys are similar to those for collecting morbidity data (see subsection A4.5.2). If, for some reason, you want to collect information on cause of death during your survey make sure you limit the information only to very common diseases such as diarrhoea and acute respiratory infection, or to any specific disease that may be causing an outbreak, for example, malaria or measles. You will need to make sure that you have very specific and locally appropriate case definitions for the causes of death.

Summary

- Mortality data should be collected using a surveillance system wherever possible. If surveillance is not possible then a cross-sectional retrospective mortality survey can be conducted alongside an anthropometric survey.
- Mortality rates give you an average rate over the recall period and cannot tell you what the mortality rate is on the day of the survey.
- Retrospective mortality surveys should employ either simple random, systematic or two-stage cluster sampling methods.
- Retrospective morality surveys should always use a separate sample from the anthropometric survey and include all households, *not* just households with children under five.
- Sample size calculations should be made for every mortality assessment in order to reduce wasting resources.
- There is no standard recall period for retrospective morality assessments. Many factors should be taken into account.
- There is currently no evidence suggesting that any of the three commonly used methods to recall mortality is better than another (the past or current census method or the previous birth history method).
- Mortality data gathered from retrospective cross-sectional surveys can very easily be biased.

Chapter C3
Producing results from mortality data

C3.1 The calculation of mortality rates from retrospective surveys

The collection of mortality data was discussed in Chapter C2. Mortality rates should be presented in the format shown in Table C3.1.

Table C3.1 Presentation of mortality rates

Crude mortality rate (CMR) (total deaths/10,000 people / day)	XX (95% confidence intervals)
Under-five mortality Rate (U5MR) (deaths in children under five/10,000 children under five/day)	XX (95% confidence intervals)

C3.1.1 Using the past and current census methods

Mortality rates for **current** census methods are calculated using the following formula:

$$\text{Mortality rate} = \frac{10,000 \text{ people}}{\text{number of recall days}} \times \frac{\text{Number of deaths during recall period}}{\text{Number of current residents} + \frac{1}{2}(\text{number of deaths during recall}) - \frac{1}{2}(\text{number of births during recall})}$$

Mortality rates for **past** census methods are calculated using the following formula:

$$\text{Mortality rate} = \frac{10,000 \text{ people}}{\text{number of recall days}} \times \frac{\text{Number of deaths during recall period}}{\text{Number of residents at start of recall} - \frac{1}{2}(\text{number of deaths during recall}) + \frac{1}{2}(\text{number of births during recall})}$$

Example C3.1: Past census method for CMR
You interviewed 900 households in a mortality survey. In total, you found 5,617 people alive at the beginning of the recall period. An estimated 67 people had died and 84 children had been born during the recall period, which was approximately 85 days long.

The calculation would be:

$$\text{Mortality rate} = \frac{10{,}000 \text{ people}}{\text{number of recall days}} \times \frac{\text{Number of deaths during recall period}}{\begin{array}{l}\text{Number of residents at start of the}\\\text{recall period}\\-\ \tfrac{1}{2}\ (\text{number of deaths during recall})\\+\ \tfrac{1}{2}\ (\text{number of births during recall})\end{array}}$$

$$= \frac{10{,}000 \text{ people}}{85 \text{ days}} \times \frac{67 \text{ deaths}}{\begin{array}{l}5{,}617 \text{ residents} - \tfrac{1}{2}\ (67 \text{ deaths})\\+\ \tfrac{1}{2}\ (84 \text{ births})\end{array}}$$

$$= 1.4 \text{ deaths} / 10{,}000 \text{ people} / \text{day}$$

The calculation for the U5MR is the same, except you only use the under-five population data.

Example C3.2: Current census method for U5MR
You interviewed 900 households in a mortality survey. In total, you found 1,124 children aged less than five years old alive in the household on the day of the survey. An estimated 45 children aged less than five years old had died and 84 children had been born in the recall period, which was approximately 87 days long.

The calculation would be:

$$\text{U5MR} = \frac{10{,}000 \text{ children} <5}{\text{number of recall days}} \times \frac{\begin{array}{l}\text{Number of deaths of children under 5}\\\text{during recall period}\end{array}}{\begin{array}{l}\text{Number of current children under 5}\\+\ \tfrac{1}{2}\ (\text{number of deaths of children}\\\text{under 5 during recall})\\-\ \tfrac{1}{2}\ (\text{number of births during recall})\end{array}}$$

$$= \frac{10{,}000 \text{ children} <5}{87 \text{ days}} \times \frac{45 \text{ deaths}}{\begin{array}{l}1{,}124 \text{ children under 5} + \tfrac{1}{2}\\(45 \text{ deaths}) - \tfrac{1}{2}\ (84 \text{ births})\end{array}}$$

$$= 4.7 \text{ deaths of children under 5} / 10{,}000 \text{ children under five/day}$$

C3.1.2 Using the previous birth history method

This methodology yields three variables per mother (see subsection C2.4.3). These are the number of:

- **children at risk**
- **new births** during recall period
- **new deaths** during recall period.

The formula to estimate U5MR is:

$$U5MR = \frac{10{,}000 \text{ children} <5}{\text{number of recall days}} \times \frac{\text{Number of deaths during recall period}}{\substack{\text{Number of children at risk} \\ + \frac{1}{2} \text{ (number of deaths during recall)} \\ - \frac{1}{2} \text{ (number of births during recall)}}}$$

Example C3.3: Use of previous birth history to calculate U5MR

You interviewed 850 mothers in a mortality survey. In total, you found that 1,445 children had been born in the last five years. These are the 'children at risk' category. An estimated 30 children aged less than five years old had died and 63 children had been born in the recall period, which was approximately 90 days long.

The calculation would be:

$$U5MR = \frac{10{,}000 \text{ children} <5}{\text{number of recall days}} \times \frac{\text{Number of deaths during recall period}}{\substack{\text{Number of current children at risk} \\ + \frac{1}{2} \text{ (number of deaths of during recall)} \\ - \frac{1}{2} \text{ (number of births during recall)}}}$$

$$= \frac{10{,}000 \text{ children} <5}{90 \text{ days}} \times \frac{30 \text{ deaths}}{\substack{1{,}445 \text{ children under 5} + \frac{1}{2} \\ (30 \text{ deaths}) - \frac{1}{2} \text{ (63 births)}}}$$

$$= 2.3 \text{ deaths} / 10{,}000 \text{ children} <5 / \text{ day}$$

C3.2 Calculating 95% confidence intervals around mortality rates

You need to calculate 95% confidence intervals around mortality rates as you do for the prevalence of malnutrition if you have sampled the survey population to obtain the mortality data.[1] The method to generate a confidence interval is

---

[1] If you have obtained mortality data from an exhaustive sample of households in an area then there is no need to calculate a confidence interval.

common to all three methods to collect mortality data (past/current census method and prior birth history).

Calculation of confidence intervals is very similar to that described for prevalence of malnutrition. Excel-based spreadsheets that do the calculation of confidence intervals from a mortality rate (currentmethod.xls, pastmethod.xls, pbh.xls) for a cluster sample survey are found on the CD-ROM found with this manual. Details about how to use the spreadsheets can be found in Appendix S7.

C3.3 Presenting age-specific mortality rates

In some situations it may be useful to look at mortality rates for different age groups in the population. If you want to do this, you will have to refine your mortality questionnaires to find out the exact age of those who died in the recall period (Chapter C2 and Appendix S6). Table C3.2 shows an example of how such data could be presented.

Table C3.2 Age- and sex-specific death rates since Eid Qurban 1379 (4–6 March 2001), Badghis Nutrition and Health Survey, March 2001

Age group (years)	Males		Females		Both sexes	
	Rate*	95% CI**	Rate	95% CI	Rate	95% CI
0–5	2.86	1.74, 4.30	2.23	1.36, 3.30	2.51	1.80, 3.47
5–14	0.20	0.01, 0.39	0.15	0.00, 0.33	0.18	0.06, 0.30
15–49	0.18	0.02, 0.34	0.47	0.11, 0.83	0.32	0.11, 0.55
50+	0.76	0.05, 1.50	0.69	0.00, 1.44	0.73	0.22, 1.26
All ages	0.69	0.41, 1.00	0.74	0.47, 1.02	0.72	0.49, 0.96

* Number of deaths / 10,000 population / day
** CI = confidence interval

Summary

- Mortality rates are expressed as the number of deaths per unit of person time.
- CMR and U5 mortality rates have different denominators.
- Mortality rates should be presented with their 95% confidence intervals.

Part D
Interpreting the findings

This section is intended to guide you through the process of interpreting the findings from your assessment. You need to interpret the findings from your causal analysis, anthropometric and mortality surveys together in order to develop appropriate recommendations. The first chapter in this section should guide you through this process. The second chapter provides some guidance on how to develop recommendations based on your interpretation of the situation. It also suggests who you need to present the information to. Finally, Chapter D outlines the most important elements of a nutrition assessment report.

Chapter D1
Interpretation of results

Once you have analysed the anthropometric and mortality data from your survey you will have results that include an estimate of the prevalence of both moderate and severe acute malnutrition and the under-five mortality rate (U5MR) and/or crude mortality rate (CMR) (Chapters B3 and C3). You will also have constructed a causal framework of malnutrition and a seasonal calendar based on the specific context of the affected population (Chapter A5). The next challenge is to draw together these three groups of information to reach judgements about the severity of the situation. This involves addressing the following three questions:

1. Is the prevalence of malnutrition 'typical' for the population in the current season?
2. Is the mortality rate 'typical' for the population in the current season?
3. How serious is the situation?

The interpretation of the results is probably the most difficult part of an emergency nutrition assessment because there is no standard method for interpreting either mortality or nutrition data, and there are many different factors to consider at the same time. However, a proper interpretation of the results is crucial if you want to make appropriate recommendations.

D1.1 Is the prevalence of malnutrition typical or not?

In theory all children under five years of age should grow at the same rate. The prevalence of wasting in the National Centre for Health Statistics (NCHS) reference population is, by definition, 2.3%. This means that the prevalence of wasting should be about 2.3% globally[1] and any prevalence higher than this should be considered abnormal.[2]

In most of the areas where emergency nutrition assessments are conducted, the prevalence of wasting is higher than 2.3% because children have inadequate diets and are exposed to poor health and care environments. This means that the prevalence of wasting in emergency-affected populations is nearly always higher than the prevalence in the NCHS reference population.

---

[1] In the reference population 15.9% of the distribution is less than −1 z score and 0.1% of the population is less than −3 z score.
[2] Note that this prevalence is for wasting only and does not include oedema.

In an emergency nutrition assessment we are looking at the difference in the population's nutrition situation as compared with a typical time. It is important to know whether or not the situation is typical for the population at the given season. Clearly, any prevalence of wasting significantly above the 2.3% level is not satisfactory and warrants further investigation. However, in some populations the prevalence of malnutrition may always be elevated above the 2.3% level and, although this is not ideal, expensive emergency programmes (for example, specialised feeding programmes) to alleviate the situation may not be justified unless the prevalence of wasting is substantially above the 2.3% seen in the reference population. Instead, it may be more useful to advocate for other types of programme which may improve the long-term situation. The prevalence of severe acute malnutrition should also be taken into account in interpreting the findings as these individuals have a particularly high mortality risk.

Geographical variation

Differences in the prevalence of malnutrition found across the world can be explained by differences in the immediate, underlying and basic causes of malnutrition (see Chapter A1). Differences in any of these factors will affect the population's nutrition status. In practice, this means we find different levels of malnutrition according to factors like agro-ecological zone and access to health facilities. If there are variations in, for example, the health environment in two otherwise similar populations, we would expect to find a difference in their nutrition status. Similarly, populations living in an area where food security is always a problem will usually have higher rates of malnutrition than a population in a food secure area (assuming other factors are equal). This means that it is important that you compare your results with results of previous surveys from the same place, otherwise differences will not be possible to interpret.

> **Example D1.1**
> In January 2002 two nutrition surveys were undertaken in different parts of Ethiopia. The results of the assessments are shown in Table D1.1. You can see that the prevalence of global acute malnutrition was much higher in Wollo than in Wolayita, even in a relatively good year (in terms of agricultural production) for both areas.

Seasonal variation

Examples of seasonal variation in acute malnutrition are found in almost every rural population. Towards the end of the hungry season, before the harvest in agricultural populations there is typically an increase in the prevalence of malnutrition. In pastoralist areas the hungry season is normally at the end of the

Table D1.1 Results of nutrition assessments undertaken in Ethiopia in January 2002

	Dessie Zuria Woreda, South Wollo, Amhara	Lowland areas of Wolayita Zone, SNNPR
Prevalence of global acute malnutrition	11.6%	4.4%
(<–2 z-scores and/or oedema)	(95% CI 8.8–15.1%)	(95% CI 2.5–6.4%)
Prevalence of severe acute malnutrition	0.8%	0.4%
(<–3 z-scores and/or oedema)	(95% CI 0.2–2.3%)	(95% CI 0.0–0.9%)

dry season when milk availability is low and animals are in poor condition. It is important to consider what is normal in terms of food security for a given season. Similarly, disease patterns differ with the seasons and some diseases (such as malaria and diarrhoea) are normally more common at certain times of year.

Example D1.2
The graph in Figure D1.1 shows the results of nutrition surveys conducted in the highland areas of Wolayita (Ethiopia) over four years in different seasons.

Population mean WHZ from the highland areas is shown for the different surveys. You can clearly see that the mean declines around April every year, and that it peaks in October. These changes in the population mean nutrition status corresponds to the agricultural calendar in Wolayita. The population harvests around September so that they are generally (except in very bad years) better off in October. The hungry season is between January and June when the population is waiting for the green maize harvest. When the sape rains come (usually in October and November), the hungry period is made better by the

Figure D1.1 The results of nutrition surveys conducted in the highland areas of Wolayita over three years in different seasons (Save the Children UK, 2000a)

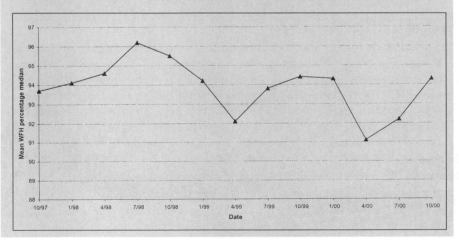

sweet potato harvest (April/May), but when the sape rains fail and there is no sweet potato harvest, there is a decline in the population's nutrition status around April.

Seasonal differences in the prevalence of malnutrition mean that when you have calculated your prevalence you need to compare them with previous survey results from the same season if possible, to find out whether or not they are normal. If you can't compare your results with earlier surveys in the same season then you need to take into account the possibility that any change in nutritional status is a typical seasonal change rather than an unusual change due to a health or food security problem.

Example D1.3
You have undertaken three surveys 30 months apart in District B and you have been asked to interpret the findings of the third survey. The main harvest in this area is normally due in April. The anthropometric results of the surveys are given in table D1.2.

Table: D1.2 Anthropometric results of surveys in District B between September 1999 and January 2001

	Global acute malnutrition (<–2 z-score and or oedema)	Severe acute malnutrition (<–3 z-score and or oedema)
September 99	7.3% (4.6–10.2%)	0.3% (0.0–0.8%)
September 00	6.8% (4.7–9.7%)	0.3% (0.1–0.7%)
March 01	13.0% (9.1–16.1%)	1.2% (0.7–1.8%)

If you looked only at the data in table D1.2 it would be difficult to properly interpret the results of the March 2001 survey. You can't tell whether or not the increase in malnutrition is due to seasonal differences – because the hungry season for this population is in March – and therefore that the prevalence is relatively normal for District B at this time of year, or, alternatively, whether the prevalence of malnutrition is particularly high because of an epidemic or a very bad year in terms of food security. If, however, you had data from another nutrition survey conducted in March then you would be able to interpret the results more easily. Without seasonal baseline data you need to collect more information on the context and causes of malnutrition in order to understand the anthropometric results of a survey.

D1.1.1 Using a local classification of malnutrition

The ideal way to assess whether or not a situation is 'typical' in terms of the prevalence of malnutrition is to compare the current situation with local baselines.[2] Ideally, baseline data provide estimates of the prevalence of malnutrition in different seasons in a 'typical' year. From this information, we can determine what is a 'typical' prevalence of malnutrition for a given time of year in a certain population. We can then decide whether or not the current nutrition status of a population is typical, or better, or worse than typical. This distinction between being concerned with the absolute level of malnutrition and the change in a population's nutrition status, helps you to plan a better intervention.

Example D1.4

In the late 1980s, Save the Children UK set up a Nutrition Surveillance Programme (NSP) to monitor the nutritional situation of the population living in the most drought-affected agricultural areas of Ethiopia. Nutrition assessments were undertaken regularly (every two to three months) in five different geographical areas for about ten years. This meant that data on the nutritional status of the population was available in both good and bad years. The results of these surveys have recently been analysed in order to produce baseline prevalences of malnutrition for the different seasons in the different areas (Table D1.3 below shows the results from two areas).[3]

Table D1.3 'Baseline' prevalences of malnutrition in North Wollo and Wag Hamra and North Shewa by season (taken from the results of the NSP surveys in 1996)

	Post-harvest (December February)	Early belg rains (March–May)	Late belg rains (June– August)	Kremt rains (September– November)
North Wollo and Wag Hamra, 1996	4.8–6.7%	5.7–7.7%	5.9–7.9%	6.9–9.0%
North Shewa	3.1–4.8%	4.2–6.0%	4.9–6.8%	4.8–6.7%

Save the Children UK closed the NSP in 2001 and only undertakes nutrition surveys on an ad hoc basis in Ethiopia now. The baseline prevalence is extremely useful when trying to decide whether or not the ad hoc survey results are 'typical' for the area or not. For example, a survey in North Wollo in the post-harvest season of 2003 estimated the prevalence of acute malnutrition at 11%.

---

[2] The Sphere Project (2004) *Humanitarian Charter and Minimum Standards in Disaster Response*.
[3] For more details on how this was done see: Save the Children UK (2004) *An analysis of Save the Children UK's Nutritional Surveillance Programme dataset in some of the most drought prone areas of Ethiopia, 1995–2001*, on the CD-ROM that accompanies this manual.

The baseline prevalence at this time of year if 4.8%–6.7%. Thus, the survey result of 11% is abnormally high and warrants further investigation and/or a response.

Information on local norms or baselines may be difficult to obtain because the data must be collected over a number of years and in different seasons, following a standard methodology so that the results from the different surveys can be compared. Usually such data are collected in nutritional surveillance systems, which are generally expensive to set up and require technical expertise. However, if the data are available it can be very useful. Section A2.2 and Appendix S1 suggest possible sources for pre-emergency anthropometric data.

Many nutrition assessments are undertaken during emergencies. This means that many agencies' survey results are not providing baseline information, but instead information about a population at a bad time. This is not true of all surveys. Some agencies undertake surveys regularly and will have data from typical years which can be considered useful as baseline data. However, you should be very careful when comparing your results with earlier results to make sure you find out what the context was in the earlier surveys. In practice, this means you have to read the previous survey report.

Comparing like with like

When you are comparing two surveys to assess the trends in malnutrition of a given population, make sure that the surveys:

1 **covered the same population** The sampling frame can vary considerably between surveys, for example, national demographic and health surveys (DHS) often exclude the most inaccessible or insecure areas, which may be the very areas where you are conducting your assessment. You should also ensure that there have not been any major migrations in or out of the survey population or significant mortality that could affect the comparability of the population. For example, excess mortality among children under five years of age distorts the age structure of the population. This affects the comparability of results between surveys. If, as a result of high mortality, the proportion of children under five in the population has fallen, then anthropometric results from this group cannot reliably be compared with a population with a normal demographic structure. This is why it is always important to check the age breakdown of your survey population (see subsection B3.4.1 for more on this).

2 **used similar methodologies** (representative sampling methods, measuring, same definitions of malnutrition (percent of the median or z-score, same age groups, etc): For example, you should not directly compare percent of the

median results with z-score results. It is often wrongly assumed that malnutrition expressed in percentage of the median or in z-scores is more or less the same. In reality, large differences can be found between the results expressed in percentage of the median and results expressed in z-scores. Typically, the prevalence of malnutrition is higher in z-scores than in percentage of the median (usually about 1.6 times as much)[4] (see also subsection B1.4.2). The differences between z-scores and percentage of the median appear to be particularly important in areas with a low prevalence of kwashiorkor, and in populations with long, thin statures (for example, Somali, Dinka and Turkana populations).

Example D1.5
A survey in 1993 in Bardera town (Somalia) and the adjacent internally displaced person (IDP) camp, found that of the 1,835 household members included in the sample survey only 8% were children under five years of age. Sixty-two per cent of the children in this age group had died in the previous nine months (so originally children under five had made up about 18% of the population). Among the children less than five years only 3% were 0–11 months old: the death rate among the infants had been especially high. Because of the high mortality rates among the younger age groups it was thought that the anthropometric survey results could not be compared to previous surveys.

Once you have obtained a relevant survey you can then start to compare your current results with earlier surveys' results and decide whether or not the nutrition of the population is typical, better or worse.

Big differences between the WHM and WHZ results can sometimes give cause for concern in survey results (see also subsections B1.4.2). These differences can be seen graphically in the shape of the distribution, which tends to be taller and narrower than the reference distribution. These differences do not usually reflect errors in the survey findings but can show that if the situation deteriorates further there could be a dramatic impact on the prevalence of malnutrition, because a high proportion of the population is at risk.

---

[4] 66 datasets from Save the Children UK anthropometric nutrition surveys were analysed to review the methods of sampling, analysis and interpretation of such surveys and their effect on the estimation of the prevalence of malnutrition. The prevalence estimated using WHZ was used as the gold standard. WHM was found to underestimate the global prevalence of malnutrition by an absolute difference of 5.2%. On average, the prevalence based on WHZ was 1.62 times that of the prevalence based on WHM. This difference was slightly less for moderate malnutrition, 4.4%, while for severe malnutrition there was little difference between the two measures, 0.8%.

Example B3.3
The results shown in Table B3.2 and Figure B3.1 come from a survey conducted in Ethiopia in an arid area inhabited by a nomadic pastoral Somali population. The survey was conducted at the end of the dry season. The population faces regular food and water shortages during the hungry season.

Table B3.2 Results of a nutrition survey in Moyale Woreda, Liban Zone

Prevalence of global acute malnutrition **(<–2 z-scores and/or oedema)**	17.1% (95% C.I. 14.3–19.8%)
Prevalence of global acute malnutrition **(<80% median and/or oedema)**	9.5% (95% C.I. 7.7–11.2%)
Prevalence of severe acute malnutrition **(<–3 z-scores and/or oedema)**	0.8% (95% C.I. 0.3–1.3%)
Prevalence of severe acute malnutrition **(<70% median and/or oedema)**	0.1% (95% C.I. 0.0–0.3%)
Crude mortality rate (CMR)	0.73/10,000/day (95% CI 0.23–1.23)
Under-five mortality rate (U5MR)	1.83/10,000/day (95% CI 1.23–2.43)

Despite the high prevalence of global acute malnutrition in z-scores, both the prevalence (z-scores and percentage of the median) of severe acute malnutrition and the mortality rates were typical. In addition, the prevalence of global acute malnutrition defined by percentage of the median and/or oedema, was not excessively high. The population was facing a difficult hungry season, but was not starving. People were not selling more livestock than usual at the end of the dry season. Camel prices were good. The situation was considered to be serious, but not critical. Thus it was decided to not implement selective feeding for the time being, but to carefully monitor the development of the rains and the food security situation over the next three months.

Note that Figure B3.1 opposite shows the distribution of global acute malnutrition defined by z-score and percent of the median for Moyale Woreda. The children between the two lines on the left of the graph are the ones defined as malnourished by the z-score but not the percent of the median. It is because this curve is so steep compared with the reference population that the difference between the prevalence rates are so high.

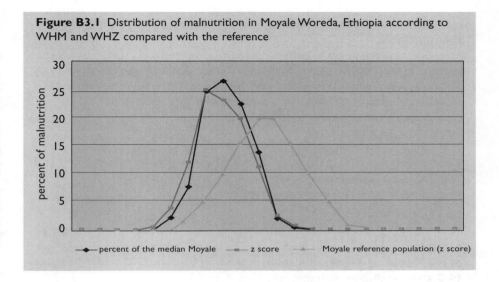

Figure B3.1 Distribution of malnutrition in Moyale Woreda, Ethiopia according to WHM and WHZ compared with the reference

Statistically comparing the level of malnutrition between two surveys

In order to see if there has been a change in the nutritional situation of a population, you need to compare the prevalence of malnutrition between two surveys. A common mistake is to report a change in nutrition status without any evaluation of whether the observed change is real, or merely a sampling artefact. These guidelines strongly recommend the use of statistics to test for a difference between the two surveys' results before any conclusions on trends are drawn from the figures presented.

The simplest way to determine whether two survey results are significantly different is to look at the CIs for each survey. If the CIs around the prevalence of malnutrition do not touch or overlap, then you can conclude there is a statistically significant difference between the two prevalence surveys. Example D1.6 shows how this can be done to compare the prevalence of vaccination coverage between two surveys conducted at the same time of year. Usually, when the CIs overlap, the difference is not statistically significant. However, in some cases even if the intervals do overlap a statistical difference may exist. Checking for this difference requires special statistical tests for which the following information is needed for each survey: the prevalence, sample size and design effect or standard error.[5] The test can then be calculated using the spreadsheet (prevdifference.xls) on the CD-ROM attached to this manual.

---

[5] These are automatically calculated in CSAMPLE within EpiInfo.

Example D1.6
The rates of measles vaccination from two different surveys are presented in Table D1.4. A measles campaign had been conducted during the period between the two surveys. Was the measles campaign successful?

Table D1.4 Results of measles vaccinations from two surveys

	April 2000 (n = 850)	April 2001 (n = 823)
Prevalence of measles vaccination *(as confirmed by card or mother)*	15.5% (95% CI 8.2–23.1%)	48.5% (95% CI 37.0–60.1%)

Yes, we can see that there has been a significant improvement in the measles vaccination rate between the two surveys because the 95% confidence intervals do not overlap. However, the rate in April 2001 was still lower than the internationally recommended rates (90%).

D1.1.2 Using a global classification of malnutrition

Global variation in the prevalence of malnutrition makes it extremely difficult to design a classification of population nutrition status which is widely applicable. What is considered a very high rate of malnutrition in one area may be 'typical' in another. Several agencies, including the WHO, have attempted to classify rates of acute malnutrition according to alert stages when the situation ceases to be typical. The WHO classification of the severity of malnutrition rates in a population is presented as an example in table D1.5 (WHO, 2000).

Table D1.5 The classification of the severity of malnutrition rates in a population according to WHO (WHO, 2000)

Severity of malnutrition	Prevalence of wasting (<–2 z-scores)
Acceptable	<5%
Poor	5–9%
Serious	10–14%
Critical	> = 15%

Unfortunately, the WHO classification has the following faults:

a) The classification does not include oedema. Oedema is a sign of severe malnutrition and must be included in any classification of acute malnutrition.
b) The classification does not take into account the severity of the causes of malnutrition and the risk which these might pose for future rates of malnutrition or mortality.
c) The highest cut-off point is a prevalence of 15 per cent less than −2 z-scores. In many parts of Africa the prevalence of acute malnutrition is above 15 per cent at the end of the hungry season, but this does not necessarily mean that the situation is so critical as to warrant an emergency nutrition response if the harvest is predicted to be normal or good.

Classifications used by other agencies (including Médecins Sans Frontières and Concern) take points (a) and (b) into account, but all the published classifications suffer from one major drawback: a tendency to over-simplify the interpretation. A classification like the one above ignores the causes of malnutrition and mortality (eg, epidemics or poor future food security), which will influence the way you interpret the anthropometric result. The classification also omits the assessment of trends in anthropometric status, which make up an important part of the interpretation of a nutrition survey.

D1.2 Is the mortality rate typical or not?

The same basic principles apply to mortality rates as to malnutrition prevalence when considering whether or not they are typical. Rates should be considered in the light of the non-emergency rates in the same population and the season.

As with malnutrition, global classifications are typically used. A crude mortality rate (CMR) of 1/10,000 per day is often taken to indicate an emergency situation (this assumes a doubling of the baseline situation in the absence of baseline data), while rates of 2/10,000 per day are taken to indicate a severe situation.[6] Under-five thresholds are 2/10,000 per day and 4/10,000 per day respectively.

Ideally, locality-specific baseline mortality rates would be available for comparison purposes because mortality rates, like malnutrition, vary according to season and area. However, in most places baseline mortality data will not be available.

The table below gives region-specific CMR and U5MR averages and emergency thresholds. The average baseline CMR for the least developed countries is 0.38 deaths/10,000 people/day. We recommend using this table as a

---

[6] For example, UN Standing Committee on Nutrition, 2004, and UNHCR, 2000

guide to classifying the stage of alert with regard to mortality, but remember that the classification is a general one and not specific to any country or season.

Table D1.6 Baseline reference mortality data by region (The Sphere Project, 2004)

Region	CMR (deaths/ 10,000/day)	CMR emergency threshold	U5MR (deaths/ 10,000 U5s/ day)	U5MR emergency threshold
Sub-Saharan Africa	0.44	0.9	1.14	2.3
Middle East and North Africa	0.16	0.3	0.36	0.7
South Asia	0.25	0.5	0.59	1.2
East Asia and Pacific	0.19	0.4	0.24	0.5
Latin America and Caribbean	0.16	0.3	0.19	0.4
Central and Eastern European Region/CIS and Baltic States	0.30	0.6	0.20	0.4
Industrialised countries	0.25	0.5	0.04	0.1
Developing countries	0.25	0.5	0.53	1.1
Least developed countries	0.38	0.8	1.03	2.1
World	0.25	0.5	0.48	1.0

Because no confidence intervals are available for the baseline rates in table D1.6, we cannot statistically compare these rates with those obtained in an emergency assessment.

D1.3 How serious is the situation?

The severity of the situation can only be judged when the three groups of information gathered in the assessment – the prevalence of malnutrition, mortality rate and causes of malnutrition are analysed together.

D1.3.1 Triangulating malnutrition, mortality and causes data

Having reached this point you should have an understanding of the most important causes of malnutrition resulting from the emergency (Chapter A5) and an understanding of whether or not the malnutrition prevalence and mortality rates are typical for the population. Now you need to assess the plausibility of your findings. This involves seeing if the results tell the same story or whether certain questions remain unanswered.

Table D1.7 gives a broad, although not comprehensive, description of the possible scenarios you may encounter during interpretation. The table should help you to decide whether your information is plausible. You should decide which situation (1–4) your assessment findings fall into, according to whether or not the mortality and malnutrition findings are typical, and then review the possible reasons for the situation in the table and compare these with your findings from the causal analysis. As was discussed in Chapter A2, your analysis of the causes of malnutrition needs to take into account ongoing interventions addressing the causes and should be focused on the gaps in intervention. Remember also that at this stage we are interested in the major causes of malnutrition resulting from the emergency, rather the ongoing problems which the community faces in non-emergency times.

Table D1.7 Possible combinations of mortality and malnutrition rates and likely causes

	High rates of mortality	Typical rates of mortality
High prevalence of malnutrition	❶ Likely causes: Acute food insecurity and failure to cope High levels of infection arising from displacement or uncontrolled epidemic Major disruption to care environment such as displaced bottle-feeding population	❷ Likely causes: Acute food insecurity Disruption to care environment resulting from damaging coping strategies No major disease outbreaks
Typical prevalence of malnutrition	❸ Likely causes: High rates of infection not typically associated with malnutrition (eg, malaria or meningitis epidemic) Mortality directly caused by conflict or acute disaster (eg, earthquake) Possible outbreaks of micro-nutrient deficiency	❹ Either no major causes of malnutrition or mortality resulting from the emergency, or causes which have yet to have an impact on malnutrition and mortality

Example of situation ❶ In Malha rural council in Darfur, Sudan, a nutrition assessment was conducted in October 2003. It showed a prevalence of global acute malnutrition of 25% and 6.1% severe acute malnutrition and an under-five mortality rate of 2.6/10,000/day. The area had been affected by drought for three consecutive years and throughout 2003 parts of North Darfur were affected by conflict, which caused considerable displacement and reduced trading opportunities and access to markets.

Example of situation ❷ In 2001 in a camp for internally displaced persons (IDPs) in Eastern Ethiopia, the IDPs had not had access to a general ration for

2–3 months and were unable to get sufficient amounts of food from other sources. The prevalence of global malnutrition was extremely high (around 30%). However, the U5MR was relatively low (1.3/10,000/day) because an international NGO was operating a very efficient therapeutic feeding programme in the camp. This programme prevented children from dying, but because the general ration was inadequate the prevalence of moderate malnutrition remained high. Moreover, many children who were discharged as normally nourished from the therapeutic programme were re-admitted a few months later as their families were unable to provide them with sufficient food to prevent them from becoming malnourished again. Recommendations from this report included an urgent need to improve the general ration.

Example of situation ❸ In Kohistan District, Afghanistan in 2001, the prevalence of acute malnutrition was estimated at 7%, which was considered typical of the area. However, the U5MR was elevated at 5.9 deaths per 10,000 per day. Members of the survey team had noticed the widespread prevalence of vitamin C deficiency disease, locally known as Seialengia (black legs). In some of the villages the deficiency disease was estimated to have affected up to 10% of the population. The team conducted a dietary investigation and found that the population had had access only to very limited sources of vitamin C in the months prior to the survey. Recommendations included vitamin C supplementation and the provision of complementary foods such as pulses, oil and blended/fortified foods for the population. It is likely that diseases other than scurvy (such as diarrhoea and acute respiratory infection – ARI) also contributed to the elevated mortality in this population.

Example of situation ❹ In Malawi in December 2001 a survey was conducted in Salima District. This showed rates of malnutrition of 9.3%, which was considered to be fairly typical for the time of year since it was the pre-harvest season. However, prices of maize were rising incredibly rapidly (much more so than usual) and becoming too expensive for people to afford. Food security assessments showed that this was likely to continue at least until the harvest. There were reports that people were starting to migrate to towns, which was normally only common in very bad years. While the nutrition assessment indicated that at the time of the survey malnutrition rates had not risen unusually high, given the prospects for the following months, rapid rises in rates of malnutrition were expected.

D1.3.2 Issues to consider during triangulation

High mortality rates and low rates of malnutrition[7]

The idea that high mortality rates can mask a deteriorating nutritional situation is widely accepted and is often referred to in nutrition assessment reports. The argument is that if the severely malnourished children die, and the survivors are the better nourished, the malnutrition rate may stabilise or even improve because of the drop-out phenomenon. This concept of 'replacement malnutrition' and the associated 'survivor bias' is often quoted when people encounter situation 3 described above.

Originally, the research to support this idea came from two cross-sectional nutrition surveys of refugees living in camps in east Sudan. The two surveys recorded similar rates of relatively high (but not critical) malnutrition over a two-month interval, but high rates of mortality had been recorded. The authors argued that the deceptive appearance of stability in nutritional status in the face of such high levels of malnutrition might be explained by ongoing nutritional deterioration ('replacement malnutrition') among surviving children.

In fact, recent research has shown that mortality rates have to be very high before this phenomenon can be observed. This is because in an emergency context infant and child deaths are not limited to the severely or moderately malnourished; deaths also occur among those who are not malnourished. A recent analysis of 266 nutrition surveys has shown that food insecurity and famine equally affect all individuals within a defined population – this means that everyone gets more wasted in the emergency (Golden and Grellety, 2002). The research found that the WFH distribution shifted to the left in emergencies, but that the shape of the distribution remained normal.

The most recent research suggests that the replacement malnutrition/survivor bias phenomenon will only be seen in populations with a very elevated CMR – maybe at a CMR of more than 10/10,000/day. Interestingly, the U5MR in the Sudanese camps in the original study was 21/10,000/day so the conclusion drawn by the authors was correct. However, you should not invoke survivor bias as the explanation for situation 3 unless mortality rates are very high.

Determining causality

It is important to remember that when you are analysing and interpreting the results of a cross-sectional survey it is not possible to prove causality. For example, if you find a high rate of malnutrition and there are reports of a measles outbreak you cannot be 100% sure that the malnutrition is due to the measles outbreak.

When you have quantitative data gathered in your survey it is possible to find out whether certain causes (such as the prevalence of diarrhoea) are associated with being malnourished, although this is relatively complex if you surveyed

---

[7] Adapted from Young H (2004) *Nutritional Assessment: progress and remaining challenges*, draft.

your population using cluster sampling and cannot easily be done on Epilnfo. But it is not possible to conclude that diarrhoea actually caused the malnutrition, only that the malnourished children had more diarrhoea. Equally, if you find that a population has abnormally high rates of diarrhoea and is also acutely food insecure you can't say that one factor is a more important cause of malnutrition than the other. You can only state that both are present and are likely to have caused malnutrition.

Levels of severe malnutrition

The prevalence of severe acute malnutrition is an important indicator because it tells you how many very malnourished children there are, and how many children are at high risk of mortality. If you have a high level of severe malnutrition and no measures in place to treat it you would expect an elevated U5MR. The proportion of wasting which is severe will increase as the prevalence of global wasting increases.

Using age breakdown of malnutrition to triangulate with causes

In Chapter B3 we stressed the importance of presenting anthropometric data by age group (subsection B3.8.2). This is because looking at the prevalence of malnutrition in different age groups can help with your interpretation of the causes of malnutrition.

Normally, the prevalence of malnutrition tends to be higher in the 6–29 month age groups than in the older age groups, because the younger groups are beginning on complementary foods or stopping breastfeeding and are more susceptible to disease. It may therefore be useful to aggregate the data into two age groups (eg, 6–29 months and 30–59 months) so that the sample of each age group is bigger and you have more statistical power to compare prevalence in the two groups (see subsection D1.1.1). Higher than normal levels of malnutrition among younger children may indicate a high burden of infection, while an equal level of malnutrition among all ages may indicate acute food insecurity.

The differences observed may promote certain programmatic responses focusing, for example, on a certain disease (such as diarrhoea). In any analysis of the age-specific prevalence of malnutrition, however, it should be remembered that the reason children aged 6–59 months are surveyed is to inform us about the situation in the whole population rather than to focus response on specific age groups of children under five.

Usually, the prevalence of malnutrition in boys and girls is similar. If there is a difference between the sexes then you need to investigate why this difference exists.

If the data do not triangulate

If when you try to bring the different types of data together you cannot make sense of the story, you should consider the following points:

1. **Bias.** Is it possible that bias has been introduced into your data? Refer back to section B2.9 and subsection B3.4.2 in consideration of this point.
2. **Time frames and populations.** Keep in mind that the anthropometric results refer to children aged 6–59 months (although they are usually thought to be a proxy for the rest of the population), the mortality results refer to everyone, and the causes of malnutrition refer to everyone but may include special investigation into groups facing special nutritional risk. The anthropometric survey measures the situation on the day of the survey, although rates of acute malnutrition at any point in time will reflect the causes of malnutrition present in the preceding period. Mortality rates refer to the recall period of the survey (not the situation on the day of the survey) and the causal analysis includes long-term as well as acute causes of malnutrition. Remember that a subsection of the population may be very severely affected by the emergency and identified in the causal analysis, but you may not pick this up in your anthropometric and mortality surveys if you did not design your surveys accordingly.
3. **Misjudging the major causes.** It is not easy to judge the extent to which a cause of malnutrition will impact on rates of acute malnutrition and mortality or how long it will be before a particular cause has an impact. Refer back to the process you went through in deciding the major causes and review whether, in retrospect, your decisions were correct.
4. **Missing information.** It is possible you failed in your causal analysis to identify a cause of malnutrition that is important. Return to the causal framework and review whether you really did fill all the information gaps.
5. **Acknowledge the inconsistency.** If after all these checks you are still not able to make sense of your data then you need to include a section in the report which states this problem and identifies the new information which would inform the findings of the assessment.

D1.3.3 Reaching conclusions

You now need to take your triangulated data and decide how serious the situation is. The extra dimension which needs to be added at this point is the seasonal calendar, explained in Chapter A5. This calendar will forecast the future and indicate whether the situation is about to get better, or worse or stay the same. This is a critical piece of information in deciding how serious the situation is.

If the causes of malnutrition or mortality are not permanent, the situation is likely to be less serious. For example, if the prevalence of malnutrition is untypically high for the time of year because of a bad year, but the harvest is due in a month and people will be able to start to eat again, then the situation will be much less serious than for a population who will not get access to a harvest for another six months. Likewise if the population has had high rates of mortality and malnutrition due to a measles outbreak but vaccination coverage is high due to a successful immunisation campaign which took place two weeks before the survey, the situation will be much less serious than if no immunisation campaign had taken place. In a situation where mortality is high and malnutrition rates are typical, the cause of mortality and whether it is permanent will be important in deciding how serious the situation is. If mortality was sudden and widespread as a result of an earthquake or massacre, and if these events were unlikely to reoccur then the situation will be less serious than if the mortality was due to an uncontrolled epidemic. Finally, if your results show that malnutrition and mortality rates are typical but that the causes of malnutrition are likely to get worse and more intense over the months following the survey then the situation could be serious.

Of course in many situations it may be impossible to predict what will happen next – eg, if insecurity is the major basic cause or if future harvests depend on a rainy season which has not yet begun. In these situations, while a spontaneous improvement may be possible, it is better to concentrate on the short term and identify how urgently assistance is required, if at all.

Summary

- There is no standard recipe for interpreting nutritional data.
- Using the global classifications for the severity of the situation can result in judgements which do not adequately take the context into account.
- In order to be able to correctly interpret anthropometric and mortality data from an emergency nutrition survey, it is necessary to:

  - determine whether the prevalence of malnutrition and the mortality rate are typical or not
  - triangulate the findings with the causes of malnutrition to decide whether the story which the data are telling seems plausible
  - decide how serious the situation is by examining your triangulated findings in the light of the prospects for improvement or deterioration gathered from your seasonal calendar.

Chapter D2
Formulating recommendations and using the information

By now you should have information on the following:

- the severity of the situation, including an understanding of the major causes of malnutrition resulting from the emergency and whether the situation is going to get better or worse. The severity of the situation dictates the urgency of the required response (see section A5.2)
- the subgroups of the population which are at greatest nutritional risk (see subsection A2.1.5)
- the chronic causes of malnutrition that need to be addressed (see section A3.1)
- the community's recommendations and understanding of their existing levels of capacity (see subsection A4.5.7)
- the feasibility of possible responses (you are unlikely to have a full understanding of this) (see subsection A4.5.8).

This information is all essential for the development of recommendations. Detailed description of emergency nutrition interventions is beyond the scope of this manual, but can be found in WHO, 2000 and 1998).

D2.1 Ten things to remember when developing recommendations

Basing recommendations on needs and rights

1. Recommendations need to be proportionate to need and should prioritise life-saving interventions. This means you need to make it clear which are the major acute causes of malnutrition and that these should be addressed as a priority before the chronic causes are addressed.
2. Recommendations need to be directly linked to your analysis of the causes of malnutrition and your judgement of the severity of the situation. You should consider recommendations which address all levels of causes (immediate, underlying and basic). It is not acceptable to recommend responses which you thought before the assessment you wanted to implement even though the assessment findings do not support this type of response.
3. Recommendations should ensure that the needs of the most affected sub-groups of the population are addressed, although this does not mean that

recommendations should necessarily include targeted interventions.

4. Recommendations should be cross-checked with the Sphere minimum standards. The Sphere standards express the rights of disaster-affected people. You should not be making recommendations which are insufficient for these rights to be achieved. For example, if rates of severe malnutrition are very high and urgent treatment is required, it would not be appropriate to recommend opening a unit in the centre of the district when you know there is no way a single unit could achieve 50% coverage, which is what is acceptable in rural areas to achieve the minimum standards (The Sphere Project, 2004).

Making recommendations time specific

5. Recommendations should include an indication of when they should be implemented to maximise their effectiveness and minimise the detrimental effect of the emergency on lives and livelihoods. They should therefore take into account the population's future needs, including immediate food prospects, potential disease outbreaks and potential changes in caring practices. Some interventions may be useless if they come at the wrong time (eg, seeds), others may cause significant hardship, malnutrition or mortality if they are late (eg, food, medical treatment).

Making recommendations feasible and building on existing capacity

6. Recommendations should always aim to build on the existing capacity within the affected population to cope with and ameliorate the effects of the crisis. This includes taking into account their recommendations for how the emergency should be dealt with.

7. Recommendations should take into account the possible harm caused by humanitarian assistance, particularly in times of conflict

8. Recommendations should be feasible. There is no point making recommendations which are impossible to implement.

9. Recommendations should be clear, where possible, about who should take responsibility for implementation.

10. Recommendations should promote the co-ordination of humanitarian agencies. In your analysis of the causes of malnutrition, you have taken into account the interventions already in place and focused on the gaps. Where possible you should take into account any interventions which you know are planned. Do not waste precious resources by making recommendations which duplicate existing or planned programmes.

D2.2 Examples of developing recommendations

Example D2.1: Nutrition assessment conducted in Binga District in Zimbabwe, March 2004: economic crisis and drought

Information required for developing recommendations	Assessment findings
Severity of the situation	Not very serious
Prevalence of global acute malnutrition <−2 z-score	2.5% (1.7–3.7)
Prevalence of severe acute malnutrition <−3 z-score	0.2 (0.0–0.8)
Crude mortality rate (CMR)	0.64/10,000/day
Under-five mortality rate (U5MR)	0.64/10,000/day
Major acute causes	Majority of poor people not able to meet their food needs due to drought, poor availability of food on the market and very high prices of available food (inflation at 600%). However, most have been receiving adequate quantities of food aid. The poor and middle wealth groups have been dependent on 75% ration for 9 months (since April 2003). High price of agricultural inputs affecting levels of production although this year 10–15% extra land has been planted. High rates of HIV and reduced capacity to pursue normal coping strategies.
Prospects	Prospects are reasonable as long as the food aid continues and the targeting of eligible groups remains accurate: 92% of children in the survey area had access to blanket supplementary feeding.
When is response needed?	No urgent response required additional to the current response.
Who is worst affected?	Poor people and social welfare cases (eg, disabled).
Long-term causes of malnutrition	Poor access to clean water and sanitation. Sporadic cases of cholera: 83% of respondents in the mortality survey did not have any form of sanitation facility.
Community recommendations and capacity	Food aid distributions should continue.
Feasibility	Programmes to address clean water and sanitation are feasible but would require funding and technical expertise.

Recommendations

- A large proportion of the population remain dependent on food aid to meet their food needs. Food aid should continue but quantities should be revised in light of the increased amount of land planted and potential alternatives to food aid. This revision should be based on a thorough food security assessment.
- Water, and especially sanitation, should be improved. This could be initiated by government authorities in collaboration with relevant NGOs and donors.

Example D2.2: Eastern Democratic Republic of Congo, Musienene health zone, May 2002: insecurity and displacement

Information required for developing recommendations	Assessment findings
Severity of the situation	Quite serious
Prevalence of global acute malnutrition <−2 z-score	8.9% (7.2–10.9)
Prevalence of severe acute malnutrition <−3 z-score	4.3% (3.0% oedema)
CMR	
U5MR	Not investigated.
Major acute causes	Poor quality diet for poor people. Poor access to health care.
Prospects	Prospects depend on the security situation. If the situation improves then malnutrition rates could decline, but kwashiorkor is likely to remain a problem, particularly seasonally.
When is response needed?	Immediately, to reduce the risk of death among people with kwashiorkor.
Who is worst affected?	Poor people and those who have been recently displaced.
Long-term causes of malnutrition	Poor access to clean water and sanitation.
Community recommendations and capacity	Any assistance needs to take into account the security situation. For example, restocking could promote looting and a deterioration in the security situation.
Feasibility	It is not feasible to put therapeutic feeding in place in areas which are inaccessible due to insecurity.

Recommendations

- Therapeutic feeding, which can be set up and closed down quickly in response to the changing security environment, should be established to treat severe malnutrition. NGOs with competence in this area of response should support this in collaboration with local authorities. General ration should not be implemented as this could destabilise the security situation.
- Feasible and appropriate food security interventions which can be targeted at poor people should be investigated to promote improved dietary quality. The Food and Agriculture Organization (FAO) and relevant NGOs should investigate options through feasibility studies.
- Supplementary feeding should not be implemented, as rates of moderate malnutrition are low.
- Ensure that drugs are available in health facilities and user fees waived for the poorest people in the community.

Example D2.3: Bangladesh, September 1998. Floods affected 75% of the country

Information required for developing recommendations	Assessment findings
Severity of the situation	**SERIOUS**
Prevalence of global acute malnutrition <–2 z-score	18.5% (16–20)
Prevalence of severe acute malnutrition <–3 z-score	2% (1.5–2.5)
	also, 5% of children reported night blindness.
CMR	Not investigated.
U5MR	
Major acute causes	Flood resulting in reduced employment opportunities, access to cash and, therefore, reduced purchasing power for food. Infection, especially diarrhoea, resulting from disruption of sanitation facilities and remaining in wet clothes and water for long periods.
Prospects	The situation will only improve when the waters recede.
When is response needed?	Immediately for relief and in the medium term for reconstruction.
Who is worst affected?	Poor people who are having to sell assets including livestock and also borrow from money lenders at high interest rates. Female- and disabled-headed households have particular difficulties in coping as their mobility is restricted.

Information required for developing recommendations	Assessment findings
Long-term causes of malnutrition	Poor access to land, limited employment opportunities.
Community recommendations and capacity	Recommended that the local representatives (eg, Chairman) should not be used as a conduit for response as they could not guarantee that the response got through. The community recommends that local NGOs, in consultation with the community and local government, implement the response.
Feasibility	Response needs to take into account limited access due to flood waters.

Recommendations

- In the immediate term, cash distribution should take place in areas where food could be purchased on the market; otherwise, food distribution with a balanced and complete household ration.
- Special effort should be made to target female- and disabled-headed households. This relief should continue until the waters recede.
- Vitamin A distribution should be initiated by the health services immediately to reduce vulnerability to infection and vitamin A deficiency.
- After the waters have receded, cash for work (and for those unable to work, cash grants) should be set up to rehabilitate the infrastructure and promote access to employment.
- Seeds should be distributed in time for the next planting, as seeds were destroyed during the flooding.
- Purification of tube-wells should be undertaken by local authorities to reduce diarrhoeal infection

Example D2.4: IDP camps in Hartishek, Ethiopia, March 2002

Information required for developing recommendations	Assessment findings
Severity of the situation	SERIOUS
Prevalence of global acute malnutrition <−2 z-score	26.6% (November 2001 was 22.0%)
Prevalence of severe acute malnutrition <−3 z-score	2.2% (November 2001 was 0.7%)
CMR U5MR	0.15/10,000/day

Information required for developing recommendations	Assessment findings
Major acute causes	The last general food distribution (GFD) was in October 2001. Food distributions were not done according to the recommended 12.5kg per household. Some households received 50kg and others none. The local administration received food for IDPs in 2002. However, the administration wants the IDP population to share the food with the local population. Until the dispute is settled, the food remains undistributed. However, TFC is operational. Water and sanitation are very poor. There is no free water delivery and no toilet facilities in the camp.
Prospects	Likely to remain the same until the general ration problems are resolved. There could be a measles outbreak in the future as there has been no measles vaccination in the last three months.
When is response needed?	Immediately
Who is worst affected?	There are no obvious groups facing nutritional risk, although there are a lot of elderly and pregnant and lactating women in the population.
Long-term causes of malnutrition	Poor access to antenatal care. Being an IDP and dependent on food aid.
Community recommendations and capacity	The IDPs have asked the government to resolve the conflict over food aid.
Feasibility	Efforts to improve water and sanitation are restricted by the absence of ground water.

Recommendations

- General rations must be reinstated immediately.
- In the absence of a general distribution, a blanket supplementary food distribution should be initiated targeting all children under five, for three months or until the general ration is provided regularly again. The blanket distribution could also target pregnant/lactating women.
- The TFC should be maintained until the situation improves.
- Safe water and improved sanitation should be provided immediately.
- All children under five should be vaccinated and provided with a vitamin A supplement.

- In the medium term, antenatal services should be provided to pregnant IDPs, and the IDPs should be supported to return home.

D2.3 What to do with the nutrition assessment report

As discussed in Chapter D1, it is extremely important that all agencies undertaking nutrition assessments in a given country share their reports with the government department responsible for emergency nutrition interventions and/ or with other agencies working in nutrition and related areas. This will enable everyone to build up a picture of the nutritional situation in the area.

Ideally, the department in the central government responsible for emergency nutrition interventions, or (in a refugee camp) the UN agency, will keep a database of nutrition reports, which can be used by any agency working in nutrition in the country. It is in the interests of all agencies to keep such a database up to date.

Survey reports should be sent to:

- the government department responsible for emergency nutrition inter-ventions at the federal/regional/district level
- MoH at the regional/district and, where appropriate, the village level
- MoA at the regional/district and, where appropriate, the village level
- planning at the regional/district level
- administration at the regional/district and village level
- NGOs working in the survey area.

If possible, inter-agency meetings should be held with the authorities and other interested agencies in the different regions, to discuss the findings of nutrition surveys, particularly the recommendations. If necessary, additions can be made to reports after these meetings.

D2.3.1 Presenting the results to the community

Finally, the results of an emergency nutrition assessment should always be presented back to the survey population. Normally this involves a trip to the district authorities.

Summary

- There is no fixed blueprint for interventions to nutrition emergencies. To try to make responses fair and effective you need to consider:
  - the severity of the situation (including an understanding of malnutrition, mortality and the major acute causes of malnutrition and whether the situation is going to get better or worse). The severity of the situation dictates the urgency of the required response
  - the sub-groups of the population which are at greatest nutritional risk
  - the chronic causes of malnutrition that need to be addressed
  - the community's recommendations and understanding of their existing levels of capacity
  - the feasibility of possible responses.
- Recommendations need to:
  - be based on need and prioritised
  - be linked to assessment findings
  - be based on Sphere standards
  - be time specific
  - be feasible
  - be built on existing capacity and community recommendations
  - promote co-ordination
  - minimise harm.
- All agencies undertaking nutrition surveys must send their results to the government, or UN agency responsible for emergency nutrition interventions, so that they can build up a central database of information on the prevalence of acute malnutrition in different parts of the country.

Chapter D3
Presenting the report

A report on the assessment should be written as soon as possible after the assessment is completed. Guidance on each section of the report is given below, followed by a model format for an assessment report.

D3.1 Brief description of the report

A brief explanation of each section of the model assessment report is given below.

Report summary
- Write the summary last, after you have finished the rest of the report.
- Ninety per cent of readers will probably only look at this section. Make sure all important information is here and is very clear. Diagrams are very useful.
- This section of the report should be short (one or two pages).
- Information should include: the area covered, the date and the objectives of the assessment, the methodology used, the main results and the recommendations.

Report introduction
- The context in which the assessment was carried out should be described. What population was surveyed, over what period and in which geographical area?
- The introduction should set out the context, so that someone who has never been to the area can understand how the surveyed community lives and what has happened to them.
- This information is mainly from secondary sources, or interviews with district officials, etc.

Objectives of the assessment
- The objectives of the assessment should be clearly stated.
- What was measured, in which population and why?

Methodology
- Describe in a straightforward way the methods employed, including sampling techniques. This is necessary so that readers can be sure of the validity of the assessment and have a clear reference for future comparison.
- Describe any problems encountered or suspected bias.

- Describe selection criteria for inclusion in the survey.
- Describe what measurements were taken, by whom and using what instruments.
- Describe how the questionnaires were designed and piloted, and how qualitative data collection was organised.

Results
- This section is mainly graphs and tables of the results gathered through the anthropometric and mortality surveys.
- A table of the distribution of the sample, according to age and sex, is required.
- All nutrition assessments should report the anthropometric statistics tables found in Chapter B3 and the mortality statistics tables in Chapter C3.

Discussion
- The discussion puts the results into context. The aim of the discussion is to explain the results (for example, prevalence of malnutrition and mortality rates) in terms of the causes of malnutrition – health, care environment and food security.
- Organise your discussion by addressing the questions in Chapter D1:
    - Is the level of malnutrition typical (referring back to previous surveys or baseline levels)?
    - Is the level of mortality typical?
    - What are the major causes of malnutrition and mortality resulting from the emergency (taking into account causes already addressed by other interventions)?
    - What are the prospects for the coming months?
    - Who is worst affected?
    - What are the chronic causes of malnutrition?
    - What does the community recommend?
    - Do the results seem plausible? Are there any unanswered questions?
- Much of the information for the discussion will come from referring back to the results section and looking at the findings in the light of your causal analysis based on key informant interviews, observations, etc.
- A diagram showing the location specific causal framework of malnutrition may be useful.

Conclusions
- This section describes the seriousness of the situation and should document the output of working through subsection D1.3.2.

Recommendations
- A report must include recommendations (see Section D2.1).

D3.2 Format for the model nutrition assessment report

Summary of the report (one to two pages only)
- area assessed
- date of assessment
- methodology employed
- main anthropometric results (prevalence of global and severe acute malnutrition in terms of z-scores and/or oedema and CIs)
- mortality rates (CMR and U5MR and CIs)
- other important results (vaccination rates, etc)
- explanation of the causes of malnutrition in the area
- recommendations, including an indication of the seriousness of the situation.

1. Introduction

1.1 Background information
Description of assessment area
- assessment area
- name of village/district/region/country
- name of nearest large town/city – administrative centre.

Population data
- number of people living in survey area
- population density
- ethnic group.

Geography of area
- town/camp/rural, etc
- altitude/mountainous/flat, etc
- total area (hectares).

Way in which people live
- information on food economy
- agriculturalists/pastoralists/agro-pastoralists/refugees/merchants, etc
- type of land farmed or animals kept.

Any important political/security information
- if refugees, how long have they been there?
- any instability in the area?

Services available
- health
- education
- markets, roads.

Assistance received by the population
- relief programmes in area
- number of people on food aid, etc
- other initiatives, particularly work of Save the Children UK in the area.

1.2 Assessment objectives
For example,
- estimate the prevalence of acute malnutrition
- estimate retrospective mortality rates
- understand the causes of malnutrition
- estimate the coverage of a feeding programme
- make recommendations for any intervention required.

2. Methodology

2.1 Assessment methodology
- General approach
- type of sampling (for example, 30×30 cluster)
- age of children measured
- number of children measured
- number of households visited for the mortality survey
- date of survey.

2.2 Sampling procedure and sample size for anthropometric data
- What was the sampling frame (including any areas excluded due to insecurity)?
- What sampling methodology did you chose? Why?
- How did you calculate the sample size? (Show the sample size calculation.)
- What population figures did you get and from whom (eg, village population figures from district council)?
- How did you calculate the sampling interval? (eg, the cumulative population was calculated and a sampling interval determined)
- How did you assign the clusters? (For example, 30 clusters were randomly selected by assigning probability proportional to population size.)
- Did you alter the method from the standard method at all (eg, increasing the number of clusters for a pastoral population)?
- Describe any changes to the selection of the clusters during the survey.

2.3 Sampling procedure and sample size for the mortality data
- What sampling methodology did you chose? Why?
- How did you calculate the sample size? (Show the sample size calculation.)

2.4 Selection of households and children
- How did you choose the households and children within a cluster?
- Where was the starting place? (Did you choose the middle of the villages? Or did you randomly chose a village within a district and start in the middle of the village?)
- How did you choose the direction to follow (eg, spin a pen)?
- Did you walk to the end of the village or district and count the houses?
- How did you choose subsequent houses?

How did you choose children within the houses?
- Did you measure all children aged 6–59 months in the houses selected?
- If age was unknown, how did you decide whether or not to measure children?
- What happened when a child was away?
- Did you measure all the children in the last house?

2.5 Training and supervision
Training
- Who was trained?
- Who did the training?
- What did the training cover (survey design, anthropometric measurements, signs and symptoms of malnutrition, data collection and interview skills)?
- Did the survey teams measure children and compare their results (inter-observer error)?

Pilot survey
- Was there a practice/pilot survey?
- Who supervised the teams during the practice survey?
- Were data collection forms piloted during the practice survey and changes made to them if necessary?

Supervision during the survey
- Who supervised the teams (a nutritionist, a nurse or someone else)?
- How many times did the supervisor visit the teams?
- Who were the team leaders? Were they experienced?

2.6 Data collected

2.6.1 Children's data
- anthropometric data
- age (proxy heights used for age)
- weight (type of scales used, precision of measurement)
- height (type of height board used, how children were measured [standing up/lying down/both], precision of measurement)
- oedema (how did you define oedema?).

Retrospective morbidity of children
- Who did you ask about the children's illnesses?
- Over what period of time did questions about illness cover?
- How did you define illness if you used a questionnaire (including description of case definitions)?

Vaccination status and coverage
- How did you check for vaccinations?
- Did you look at maternal and child health (MCH) cards?

Feeding programme coverage
- How did you assess this?
- What did you do if you found a malnourished child who was not registered?

2.6.2 Mortality data
- Retrospective mortality (under five and total population)
- What type of questionnaire/recall method did you use to estimate mortality rates?
- In which households did you use the mortality questionnaires?
- Over what period of time did you estimate mortality (number of months)? How long was the recall period?
- Did you categorise deaths by age?
- Did you record cause of death? How did you define causes?

2.6.3 Causes data
- Secondary data on the causes of malnutrition
- What sources did you get your secondary data from?

Primary data on the causes of malnutrition
- How were the key informant and focus group discussion topics developed?
- Were the questions adjusted after the practice survey?
- What kind of data did you collect in the key informant interviews?

- Who was asked the questions (community leaders, women, etc)?
- Did you visit any government officials? Who? For what information? Any other NGOs?
- What observations were made?
- Did you use a household questionnaire?
- How were the household questionnaires developed?
- Were the questionnaires adjusted after the practice survey?
- What kind of data did you collect in the household questionnaires?
- Who was asked the questions to (how many households, which people in the household)?

2.7 Data analysis
- How did you analyse the data (qualitative and quantitative)?
- What type of computer programme did you use or did you do it by hand?

3. Results

3.1 Anthropometric results: children
- Definitions of acute malnutrition should be given (eg, global acute malnutrition is defined as <−2 z-scores weight-for-height and/or oedema, severe acute malnutrition is defined as <−3z-scores weight-for-height and/or oedema).

Distribution of age and sex of sample

	Boys no.	%	Girls no.	%	Total no.	%	Ratio boy:girl
6–17 months							
18–29 months							
30–41 months							
42–53 months							
54–59 months							
Total							

Prevalence of acute malnutrition[1] based on weight-for-height z-scores and/or oedema

	6–59 months n =
Prevalence of global malnutrition **(< –2 z-score and/or oedema)**	XX % (95% CI XX–XX)
Prevalence of moderate malnutrition **(< –2 z-score and >= –3 z-score)**	XX % (95% CI XX–XX)
Prevalence of severe malnutrition **(< –3 z-score and/or oedema)**	XX % (95% CI XX–XX)

The prevalence of oedema is XX%
Standard error is XX
Design effect is XX

Prevalence of acute malnutrition by age based on weight-for-height z-scores and/or oedema

		Severe wasting (< –3 z-score)		Moderate wasting (>= –3 and < –2 z-score)		Normal (> = –2 z-score)		Oedema	
Age (mths)	Total no.	No.	%	No.	%	No.	%	No.	%
6–17									
18–29									
30–41									
42–53									
54–59									
Total									

Prevalence of acute malnutrition by sex based on weight-for-height z-scores and/or oedema

	Boys n =	Girls n =
Prevalence of global malnutrition **(< –2 z-score and/or oedema)**	XX % (95% CI XX–XX)	XX % (95% CI XX–XX)
Prevalence of moderate malnutrition **(< –2 z-score and >= –3 z-score)**	XX % (95% CI XX–XX)	XX % (95% CI XX–XX)
Prevalence of severe malnutrition **(< –3 z-score and/or oedema)**	XX % (95% CI XX–XX)	XX % (95% CI XX–XX)

The prevalence of oedema is XX%

---

[1] Underweight and stunting can be reported if age data are reliable and the data will be used for decision-making.

Distribution of acute malnutrition and oedema based on weight-for-height z-scores

	< –2 z-score	>= –2 z-score
Oedema present	Marasmic kwashiorkor	Kwashiorkor
	XX	XX
	(XX%)	(XX%)
Oedema absent	Marasmic	Normal
	XX	XX
	(XX%)	(XX%)

Prevalence of acute malnutrition based on the percentage of the median and/or oedema

	6–59 months n =
Prevalence of global acute malnutrition **(<80% and/or oedema)**	XX % (95% CI XX–XX)
Prevalence of moderate acute malnutrition **(<80% and >= 70%)**	XX % (95% CI XX–XX)
Prevalence of severe acute malnutrition **(<70% and/or oedema)**	XX % (95% CI XX–XX)

The prevalence of oedema is XX%

Prevalence of malnutrition by age, based on weight-for-height percentage of the median and/or oedema

Age (mths)	Total no.	Severe wasting (<70% median)		Moderate wasting (>= 70% and <80% median)		Normal (> = 80% median)		Oedema	
		No.	%	No.	%	No.	%	No.	%
6–17									
18–29									
30–41									
42–53									
54–59									
Total									

3.2 Mortality results (retrospective over x months prior to interview)

Mortality rates

CMR (total deaths/10,000 people / day)	(95% CIs)

U5MR (deaths in children under five/10,000 children under five / day)	(95% CIs)

Report the main causes of death as given by the MoH and the community leaders.

3.3 Children's morbidity

If you have collected data on children's morbidity using a household questionnaire then you should present it in the format shown below.

Prevalence of reported illness in children in the two weeks prior to interview (n =)

	6–59 months
Prevalence of reported illness	XX% (95% CI XX–XX)

3.4 Vaccination results

Symptom breakdown in the children in the two weeks prior to interview (n =)

	6–59 months
Diarrhoea	XX% (95% CI XX–XX)
Cough	XX% (95% CI XX–XX)
Fever	XX% (95% CI XX–XX)
Measles	XX% (95% CI XX–XX)
Other	XX% (95% CI XX–XX)

Vaccination coverage: BCG vaccination for 6–59 months and measles for 9–59 months

	BCG **n = XX**	**Measles** **(with card)** **n = XX**	**Measles** **(with card or confirmation** **from mother)**
YES	XX% (95% CI XX–XX)	XX% (95% CI XX–XX)	XX% (95% CI XX–XX)

3.5 Programme coverage

Programme type	
Supplementary feeding programme coverage	% (95% CI)
Therapeutic feeding programme coverage	% (95% CI)

(This table should be adjusted if CSAS method is used.)

Data on the causes of malnutrition (other than those above)
- Leave this for the discussion

4. Discussion

4.1 Nutritional status
- Discuss sample sex ratio – any bias? If so, explain why you think there is bias.
- State the prevalence of acute malnutrition.
- If previous survey results are available, how do these results compare with before, or with other areas nearby?
- How does the prevalence compare with national benchmarks of malnutrition?
- Is the prevalence of malnutrition typical or not?

4.2 Mortality
- Do you suspect any bias in the findings?
- What is the mortality rate?
- If previous survey results are available, how do these results compare with before, or with other areas nearby?
- How do the rates compare with baseline rates?
- Is the mortality rate typical or not?

4.3 Causes of malnutrition
- What are the major causes of malnutrition resulting from the emergency? Where possible, state the causes of mortality (taking into account causes already addressed by other interventions). Consider immediate, underlying and basic causes.
- What are the prospects for the coming months? Will the situation get better or worse (refer to seasonal changes, etc)?
- Who is worst affected?
- What are the chronic causes of malnutrition?
- What does the community recommend?
- Do the results seem plausible? If not, what are the unanswered questions?
- A diagram to show the causal framework of malnutrition may be useful.

4.4 Programme coverage

- Give the rate of coverage for any supplementary or therapeutic feeding programmes.
- Explain the rates (good/bad/why).
- Given the prevalence of malnutrition found, how many children should be enrolled?

5. Conclusions

- State your overall conclusions on the severity of the situation and the urgency of the response required.

6. Recommendations and priorities

- Remember to prioritise recommendations and try to give a timescale which would be appropriate (eg, immediate, medium term or longer term).

Future nutrition monitoring

- Is it necessary to carry out another nutrition survey in this area in the near future? Who should do it? Should there be any changes to the survey methodology? When should the survey take place?
- Should there be food security indicator monitoring in this area? Who should do it?

7. References

List all secondary sources to which you have referred in the text.

8. Annex

- Maps of area
- Questionnaires
- List of clusters (village and district names).

Section E
Fifteen practical steps for conducting an assessment

This chapter will describe the 15 practical steps for undertaking a nutrition assessment. Some of the steps have been described in detail earlier in the manual and so will only be referred to briefly here. Other steps have not been discussed yet and will be described here in full.

There will, of course, be overlap between these steps, particularly the first four steps, and so the exact order in which you undertake these activities may not be the same as the order described here. Steps 1–3, 6–9 and 15 will probably take place in the office. The remaining steps will normally take place in the field.

Step 1: Decide whether or not an assessment is necessary

The decision to undertake a nutrition assessment will usually be made in conjunction with the government and other partner agencies. The actual decision-making process will depend on local circumstances and relationships. It is, however, always important to share information about when and where you plan to undertake a nutrition assessment, to prevent repetition and overlap of assessments.

Conducting a nutrition assessment is expensive and time consuming, so before starting you should consider the following points.

* Are the results crucial for decision making? If a population's needs are obvious, immediate programme implementation is the first priority. A nutrition assessment can be carried out later. For example, if there has been a natural disaster, such as an earthquake or landslide, and it is clear that the population's main food source has been destroyed, it may not be necessary to undertake a nutrition assessment. Similarly, if another agency has recently carried out a nutrition assessment in the same area then it should not be necessary to repeat the process.
* The assessment results must be used to inform action. There is no point undertaking a nutrition assessment when you know that a response will not be possible. Before undertaking the assessment you should ensure that a response is possible, if one is needed. It should be noted that the Sphere minimum standards require that a nutrition assessment is conducted if a targeted feeding programme is implemented.

- Is the affected population accessible? Insecurity or geographical constraints may result in limited access to the population of interest. If this is extreme, an assessment cannot be conducted.

You should not undertake a nutrition assessment unless these three prerequisites are fulfilled.[1]

Step 2: Define assessment objectives

Before starting any nutrition assessment you must be clear about your objectives. Precise and clear objectives will make it much easier for your team, the assessment population and donors to understand what you are trying achieve.

If the assessment is undertaken in an emergency situation, the nutrition information should help the agency to:

- estimate the prevalence of acute malnutrition in children aged 6–59 months
- understand the causes of malnutrition
- if necessary, make recommendations about suitable interventions.

Alternatively, if the assessment is undertaken during a good or normal time, then the data can be used to establish a baseline from which changes in nutritional status can be monitored over time.

Undertaking a nutrition assessment provides an ideal opportunity for agencies to see a population they are assisting, or planning to assist. It is useful to collect additional information on the population, such as mortality, immunisation and nutrition programme coverage data where no routine surveillance information is available. This can help inform interventions. Thus, many nutrition assessments have additional objectives which include estimating:

- the prevalence of measles vaccination and the rate of vitamin A supplementation
- impact and coverage of feeding programmes
- mortality rates.

Step 3: Define geographic target area and population group

You need to decide in which area the assessment should be conducted, and which population groups you will assess. In most cases, the area chosen will correspond to one or more administrative areas (for example, a district). The

---

[1] Sometimes it may be difficult to fulfil the second requirement (ie, make sure that a response will be possible) if the results are going to be used to lobby for a response.

assessment must be conducted in an area where the whole population has a similar nutritional situation. Remember that if you conduct an assessment of an area with two very different agro-ecological zones or FEZs, the results will be averaged over the two zones and will mask any differences that exist. You can only resolve this by undertaking two separate assessments, but this is costly (see Section B2.2).

You also need to decide at this point what age group to measure. As stated in Chapter B1, anthropometric assessments are usually carried out among children aged 6–59 months. Young infants may be included if you suspect that there is an acute nutritional problem in this group (Section B1.8).

In some situations, an anthropometric assessment can be conducted among adults or adolescents, but remember these assessments are much harder to undertake and you should seek advice from technical experts before proceeding with this (see Section B1.7).

Step 4: Meet the community leaders and local authorities

It is absolutely essential to meet the community leaders and local authorities before trying to start a nutrition assessment. During your visit you should:

- make sure the community fully understands the objectives of the assessment. If the population does not understand why you are doing an assessment, you may not be able to get co-operation during the assessment's implementation
- agree the dates of the actual assessment with the community leaders and local authorities
- obtain information on population figures (particularly at village or camp level)
- obtain information on security in, and access to, the assessment area.
- obtain a map of the area in order to plan the assessment
- obtain letters of permission from the local authorities, addressed to the district or village leaders, stating that you will be visiting. The letters should explain why you are conducting an assessment and ask for the population's co-operation.

Step 5: Determine timing of the assessment

The exact dates of the assessment should be chosen with the help of community leaders and local authorities in order to avoid the assessment conflicting with market days, local celebrations, food distribution days, vaccination campaigns, or other times when people may be absent. It is important to take the agricultural calendar into consideration, because women and children may be in the fields for most of the day during certain seasons.

The assessment schedule should allocate time for preparation and literature review, training, pilot testing, community mobilisation, data collection, analysis and reporting.

Step 6: Select sampling methods and clusters (if required)

Once you have decided what population group in which geographical area you want to assess, you can decide on your sampling method and, if necessary, select the clusters. This process is described fully in Chapter B2. Remember to select extra clusters if you are in an insecure area or in a place where the population is scattered over a wide area.

Don't forget to calculate the sample size separately for both mortality and anthropometric data.

Step 7: Gather all available secondary information

Before starting the assessment, all available secondary information should be collected, as discussed in Chapter A2. This includes population characteristics and figures, previous assessments, health statistics, food security information, etc. This is a critical step in the analysis of the causes of malnutrition and leads to the development of the pre-assessment causal analysis. Once you establish what information is available, you will know what extra information you need to obtain during the assessment. Only then you can start to design your questionnaires and plan your key informant interviews.

Step 8: Decide what information to collect and design questionnaires and surveyor's manual

The information you collect must correspond to the objectives of the assessment. You should also devise a plan of analysis prior to the data collection to ensure the validity of the questions and to get the responses in a format that is easy to use during data entry and analysis.

Remember that in order to plan an intervention to a nutrition crisis properly, information on the likely causes of malnutrition must be available at the end of any nutrition assessment (see Chapters A1 to A5).

E1.8.1 Children's anthropometric data

When you are estimating the prevalence of acute malnutrition in children aged 6–59 months, the following data should always be collected:

- age, in months (from a known date of birth or based on an estimate derived from a calendar of local events)
- sex
- weight in kilograms (to the nearest 100g)
- height in centimetres (to the nearest millimetre if possible, otherwise to the nearest half centimetre)
- presence of oedema.

According to specific assessment objectives, other data is optional:
- measles immunisation status (and possibly anti-tuberculosis vaccination – BCG)
- vitamin supplementation status, especially vitamin A
- morbidity
- nutrition programme coverage
- MUAC (to the nearest 1mm).

An example of a standard children's anthropometric questionnaire is given in Section S6.1, Appendix S6.

E1.8.2 Mortality data

It is relatively easy to couple a mortality survey with an anthropometric survey, but remember that different households will be included in the different assessments. An anthropometric survey only includes households with children aged 6–59 months, whereas a mortality survey must include all households. You need to decide which recall/questionnaire method to use to collect mortality data (see Chapter C2).

Examples of standard mortality questionnaires are given in Section S6.2, Appendix S6.

E1.8.3 Other data

A variety of methods can be used to collect extra data. This includes using a household economy approach (HEA), household questionnaires, key informant interviews, market assessments and observation. These methods are all described in Chapter A4.

If you have decided to collect food security information during the nutrition assessment then it is important to have someone familiar with food security information working with you. This person will be responsible for helping the team plan the key informant discussions and, if necessary, design the household questionnaires.

E1.8.4 Surveyor's manual

If questionnaires are complicated they should be accompanied by a surveyor's manual containing details on how each question should be asked and recorded. A surveyor's manual is intended as a guide for nutrition assessment teams working in the field. However, they are optional – you only need one if you think the team might need some clarification in the field.

An example of a surveyor's manual for standard anthropometric and mortality questionnaires is given in Section S8.1, Appendix S8.

E1.8.5 Translate the questionnaires into the local language

If you have designed your questionnaires in English, or another non-local language, then it may be necessary to translate the questionnaires into the local language. This is time consuming, but useful and necessary to ensure all the team members understand the questionnaire. In turn, this should mean that all the teams are asking the assessment population the same questions.

Step 9: Obtain and prepare equipment

Measuring material, scales and height boards should be in perfect condition and regularly tested for accuracy. For example, during an assessment, scales should be checked each day against a known ten kilogram weight. If the measure does not match the weight, the scales should be discarded or the springs must be changed.

A list should be made of required equipment, which should include the transport facilities, fuel, paper and pens needed per day, etc. An example of a list of materials needed for an assessment is given in Section S8.2, Appendix S8. Information about minimum standards for anthropometric measuring equipment can be found in Appendix S2.

Copies of questionnaires, absentee forms and forms for referral of moderately or severely malnourished cases to supplementary feeding and therapeutic feeding programmes (if they exist), should be prepared.

Step 10: Field test the questionnaires

Once you have designed your questionnaire and your questions for key informant interviews and focus group discussion you need to field test them. This is done to ensure there are no errors, and that the population can easily understand and respond to the questions. There is no standard method for field testing. Normally you would try out questionnaires on about ten households or interview checklists on a couple of focus groups.

After the field testing you should alter your questions as necessary. For example, if the respondents had difficulty understanding a particular question, you need to change the language of the question or shift the emphasis of the question.

Field testing should not take place in a location where the proper assessment will take place, but in a similar community. For example, you could field test in a neighbouring village that has not been selected during the cluster sampling. Do not forget to get a permission letter from local authorities, even for field testing.

It should be noted that field testing questions forms a separate activity to pilot testing the assessment method, which takes place during team member training (described in Step 12).

Step 11: Select the assessment team

Assessment teams usually consist of three people: two to undertake the measurements and one writer/supervisor. The supervisor is responsible for the quality and reliability of the data collected. It is often also useful to have a respected community member on the team. This person can introduce the assessment team to the population and assist in guiding the team around the location. The community member is additional to the core (trained) three-person team. In some cases it is also necessary to have a translator on the team.

The team can be composed of health workers, but team members do not have to be health professionals. Anyone from the community can be selected and trained as long as they are able-bodied (there is normally a lot of walking involved) and have a relatively high educational level. They must be able to read and write fluently (we suggest employing people with Grade 10 education or more). Women have more experience of dealing with young children and so are very useful members of an assessment team.

Two to six teams may be needed according to the number of households to be visited and the size and accessibility of the area covered. Obviously, if you are in a great hurry to get the results, it is better to have more teams. However, the more teams you have the larger the variation in the precision of the results. Moreover, it is difficult to supervise and organise (logistically) a larger number of teams.

In general, it is very useful to have an assessment supervisor as well as the team supervisors. This person should be experienced in undertaking nutrition assessments, training and managing logistics and people. The assessment supervisor will be responsible for training the team members. In addition he or she will visit the teams when they are in the field and check that they are undertaking the assessment properly.

Step 12: Train assessment team members

The training of assessment team members is a key step for the proper implementation of a nutrition assessment. All members should undergo the same training, whatever their former experience, to ensure standardisation of methods. The training usually takes two or three days and should include:

- a clear explanation of the objectives of the assessment
- an explanation of the sampling method. This should stress the rationale and the importance of representativeness
- a demonstration and practice of weight and height measurements. Each measurer should practise ten to twenty height and weight measurements and an oedema assessment. Appendix S3 describes a method for helping team members to standardise their measurements. The purpose of the standard-isation exercise is to detect and correct errors in measurement techniques prior to the assessment
- an explanation of the questionnaire and questions for discussion in order to verify the formulation of the questions. Role-play exercises are useful for this. If you have prepared a surveyor's manual then you should also explain and test this
- a pilot assessment in the field. This is the time to test all parts of the assessment under realistic conditions. Make sure you visit a location that will not be in the real assessment but which is similar to the assessment site. Data collected during the pilot assessment should not be used in the analysis of the results.

A pilot assessment is different from field testing the questionnaire as it is intended to ensure you test all the parts of an assessment, including:

- the sampling procedure. This means the team will practise selecting the first house and children of the right age
- how to take and record measurements correctly. This means the team will practise distributing measuring tasks between them
- how to conduct interviews. The teams will practise using the questionnaire and surveyor's manual, and conducting focus group interviews. If necessary, the questions and assessment manual can be changed after the pilot visit
- how to organise the equipment logistically (transport and care of equipment).

At the end of the pilot assessment, the team members and assessment supervisor will have an idea about how long the questionnaires and measurements will take for each child and how long the key informant discussion will take. This information will help you calculate how many children you can expect to measure each day during the real assessment, and so will help you plan your assessment timetable.

Step 13: Implement the assessment

There are several ways to improve the quality of the data collected during a nutrition assessment.

- Ensure that errors in the field are minimised by using good-quality equipment which is regularly calibrated.
- Check the forms for blank entries at the end of each day to make sure no data is left out. The team supervisor should review all questionnaires before leaving an area in order to make sure no pieces of data have been left out. If there are any problems, the team can return to the household.
- Ensure regular supervision of assessment teams by the assessment supervisor. In particular, the assessment supervisor should check for cases of oedema. If team members are not properly trained it is easy for them to mistake a 'fat' child for one with oedema (particularly with younger children). Assessment supervisors should look out for teams that are reporting an excessive amount of oedema and should visit some of these children to cross-check.
- Do not overwork your teams. When people are tired – and nutrition assessments can be very tiring because of all the walking involved – they make mistakes. Make sure the team has enough supplies to keep them going.

Step 14: Analyse and interpret your findings during the assessment

Do not wait until you have completed your fieldwork before beginning to analyse and understand your findings; during fieldwork you can learn as you go. Record important points in a notebook as soon as you can. Include observations, ideas or hunches. Remember to record the reasons behind them. Label notes with the date, location and name(s) of relevant people. For more information see Chapters A4 and A5.

The team should regularly discuss their findings together. This may bring out important points or indicate necessary changes in the assessment methods.

If possible, at each household, the team supervisor should calculate the WHM for each child and classify their nutrition status. If the supervisor finds a malnourished child, he or she should refer the child to the nearest facility, where possible. Ideally this will be a therapeutic or supplementary feeding programme. Obviously, logistical and security constraints have to be taken into account.

At the end of the data collection process, the team should work together to analyse the results and interpret the findings.

Step 15: Write the report

The final part of a nutrition assessment is the report writing. The results of the assessment should be presented in a standardised format so that different assessments can be compared. This is explained further in Chapter D3.

Agencies must produce their reports in a timely fashion. The results of an emergency assessment must be released and disseminated as soon as possible to prevent any delay in the intervention. Draft reports for emergency nutrition assessments should be available within ten days of the assessment being completed and the final report available within three weeks. Baseline assessment reports may not be needed so rapidly.

Summary

There are 15 practical steps for conducting an assessment:

1. Decide whether or not an assessment is necessary.
2. Define assessment objectives.
3. Define geographic target area and population group.
4. Meet the community leaders and local authorities.
5. Determine timing of the assessment.
6. Select sampling method and clusters (if required).
7. Gather all available secondary information.
8. Decide what information to collect and design questionnaires and surveyor's manual.
9. Obtain and prepare equipment.
10. Field test the questionnaires.
11. Select the assessment team.
12. Train assessment team members.
13. Implement the assessment.
14. Analyse and interpret your findings during the assessment.
15. Write the report.

Part F
Evaluating programme impact and assessing coverage

Nutrition assessments often have the dual purpose of measuring the level of malnutrition and estimating the impact of an intervention. Using assessments in this way is discussed in the first chapter of this section. The second chapter deals specifically with measuring the coverage of a feeding programme and presents possible methods to do this effectively. Coverage is a measure of programme impact, as it indicates the proportion of the eligible population who have accessed the programme.

Chapter F1
Monitoring and evaluating emergency nutrition programmes

Nutrition survey results, specifically anthropometric data, may be used to assess the impact of nutrition programmes such as general food distributions (GFDs), supplementary feeding programmes (SFPs) and therapeutic feeding programmes (TFPs).[1] This is an essential part of the management of such programmes: survey results should be used to adjust programmes, particularly if the objective of a programme is to improve the population's nutrition status. Nevertheless, an improvement or deterioration in nutrition status normally *cannot* just be attributed to the quality of the nutrition programmes implemented.

Three important questions need to be asked when assessing nutrition programmes:

- What is the impact of the programme on the nutrition status of the whole area within which the programme operates?
- What is the impact of the programme on the nutrition status of those households receiving assistance, ie, the beneficiaries?
- Should the programme be closed or altered?

The discussion below will focus on how nutrition data can be used to answer these questions. The importance of non-anthropometric data for programme monitoring and evaluating will also be discussed.

F1.1 Non-anthropometric data needed to monitor and evaluate nutrition interventions

Before discussing how anthropometric survey data can be used to monitor and evaluate nutrition interventions, we need to consider what other data is necessary. You need other, non-anthropometric data to evaluate a nutrition (or food security or health) programme because you need to be able to explain why there has been

---

[1] Nutrition surveys are also used to assess food security interventions and health or sanitation programmes. However, this is more complex because such interventions do not always directly impact on nutrition status and so it is harder to monitor and evaluate them on the basis of anthropometric data.

an improvement or deterioration in nutrition status. For example, you need to know whether it was the nutrition intervention that improved the situation, or some other factor.

Many factors contribute to a change in a population's nutritional status, as has been described in Chapters A1 to A5. Any of the underlying and basic causal factors that determine malnutrition could have changed.

For example, households' access to food could have increased because of a harvest, a decrease in cereal market prices, an increase in demand for labour, or other income-generating activities. Unfortunately, this normally means you cannot be sure exactly how useful the nutrition intervention was – unless absolutely no other factors have changed between the two surveys. The only way to deal with this problem is to try to find out what other factors have changed, and then try to work out how important the nutrition programme was.

> **Example F1.1**
> You undertake a follow-up nutrition survey in an agricultural district and find there has been a significant decrease in malnutrition since a food-for-work programme started in the area. How can you tell whether or not this is due to the programme or other factors? You need to find out what other factors have also changed through carrying out a HEA assessment and/or discussions with key informants or through community or household questionnaires.

If a continuing deterioration in nutrition status is found in an area after a relief food programme has been implemented, then you should consider the following factors:

- Was the beneficiary number adequate?
- Was the ration size adequate?
- Was the food delivered frequently enough?
- Does a health problem exist? Should a health intervention be considered?
- Was the targeting system properly implemented?
- Are the young children receiving their fair share of the food?

F1.2 How can you measure the impact of a programme on the whole population?

Repeated cross-sectional surveys are a very useful way to assess the impact of a programme on the whole area. Cluster surveys can be made at the start of an intervention and then a few months later to assess the nutrition status of the whole population. Subsection D1.1.1 describes how to test whether differences between surveys are significant or not.

Frequently, programmes are set up to address a short-term period of hunger – eg, in a year where conflict or drought has been particularly bad. These programmes are then closed when the situation improves. Nutrition assessments are conducted at the beginning and the end. Reduction in the prevalence of malnutrition during this period would be expected regardless of any intervention since the end survey is likely to be conducted after the harvest or when people have recovered from the insecurity. This means it is not appropriate to attribute improvement to the intervention alone. You must also acknowledge that some of the major causes of malnutrition have been addressed spontaneously and that this will play a major part in the reduction in malnutrition (see Example F1.2).

Example F1.2

In Gola Oda in Ethiopia rates of malnutrition were assessed; the results are shown in the Table F1.1. From January 2003 a general ration was in place and from April 2003 supplementary and therapeutic feeding, which achieved reasonable coverage, was implemented. While the rates of malnutrition declined significantly by the end of the project period, the short-maturing maize was harvested in September and the long-maturing sorghum was harvested in December which would have also contributed to reductions in malnutrition.

Table F1.1 Rates of malnutrition in Gola Oda, Ethiopia

	Global acute malnutrition (< –2 z-score)	Severe acute malnutrition (< –3 z score and /or oedema)
November 2002	15%	1.1%
	95% CI (11.5–18.5%)	95% CI (0.4–1.8%)
December 2003	6.3%	0.5%
	95% CI (4.1–8.5%)	95% CI (0.1–0.9%

F1.3 How can you measure the impact of the programme on the beneficiaries?

You cannot measure the impact of a programme only on the beneficiaries, using repeated cluster surveys, unless everyone in the population was a beneficiary. In order to measure the impact on individuals receiving food, for example in an SFP, it is necessary to follow up those individuals directly. This means each child in an SFP should initially be registered, weighed and measured, and then s/he should be longitudinally measured over time.[2]

---

[2] The process of monitoring individuals in SFP programmes, and also the progress of the whole SFP, is beyond the scope of this manual. Information on this is available from WHO (2000) and Médecins Sans Frontières (1995).

The same is true for households. If you want to measure the change in nutrition status only in households included in food distributions, then you would have to set up a longitudinal survey that looked specifically at this group. A description of such a survey is beyond the scope of this manual.

Chapter F2
Measuring programme coverage

Knowing programme coverage is important for monitoring and evaluating selective feeding programmes. Unless high levels of coverage can be achieved, a programme will not have a significant impact on the population. Coverage data are often required for donors. Coverage data are also useful to help project staff find out how well a project is doing and whether or not the project is meeting, or will meet, its objectives.

This chapter outlines different approaches to estimating programme coverage and discusses their shortcomings. Recommendations are given about which method to use, and when. Interpretation of coverage figures is also discussed.

F2.1 Standard approaches to assessing programme coverage

Currently, standard approaches to assessing coverage of SFPs and TFPs involve making use of anthropometric surveys either *directly*, using the survey data, or *indirectly*, using survey data, programme enrolment data and population estimates. Note that if, during the survey, you find a malnourished child who is not enrolled on the programme then you should refer her/him to the programme immediately.

F2.1.1 Direct method to assess coverage

The direct method involves adding a question to the anthropometric question-naire about whether or not a child is currently enrolled in a feeding programme (Table F2.1 gives an example of this question). This is probably the most commonly used method to assess coverage. An example of an anthropometric questionnaire with these questions added is given in Section S6.1, Appendix S6.

Table F2.1 Example of a coverage question to be added to an anthropometric questionnaire

Is (name of child) registered in the SFP or TFP now?	0	=	no
	1	=	SFP
	2	=	TFP

Coverage is then estimated using the following equation:

$$\text{Coverage} = 100 \times \frac{\text{Number of eligible children found attending the programme during the survey}}{\text{Number of eligible children found during the survey}}$$

An eligible child is defined as a child who should be enrolled in the programme. For example, a moderately malnourished child WHM <80% and WHM > = 70%) should be enrolled for an SFP and hence would be eligible for that type of programme. A severely malnourished child (WHM<70% and/or oedema) should be enrolled in a TFP and hence would be eligible for that type of programme.

Example F2.1

Imagine there is a supplementary feeding programme for all moderately malnourished children and a therapeutic feeding programme for the severely malnourished children in District A. During the nutrition survey, you find 23 moderately malnourished children who are registered on the SFP and 107 moderately malnourished children who are not registered in the programme. You find nine severely malnourished children, of whom two are registered on the TFP. You measure a total of 908 children. What are the programme's coverage rates as estimated by the direct method?

$$\text{SFP coverage} = 100 \times \frac{23}{23+107}$$

$$= 17.7\%$$

$$\text{TFP coverage} = 100 \times \frac{2}{9}$$

$$= 22\%$$

You should always calculate CIs for your estimate of coverage. The method to do this is the same as for the prevalence of malnutrition, outlined in Appendix S7. The sample size (or number of children in each cluster) should be taken as the number of malnourished (or eligible) children in the survey, not the sample size of all children in the survey.

F2.1.2 The indirect method for assessing coverage

The indirect method involves comparing the number of malnourished children estimated to exist in a population through a nutrition survey with the actual number of children attending the programme. There is no need to add a question to the anthropometric questionnaire. This method is usually less accurate than the direct method because it requires relatively up-to-date information on population figures.

Coverage is estimated using the following equation:

$$\text{Coverage} = 100 \times \frac{\text{Number of children attending the feeding programme}}{\substack{\text{Estimated prevalence of malnutrition} \times \\ \text{estimated number of children in the population}}}$$

It is important that you always compare like with like. You must always take children in the same age group. For example, if children are only eligible for feeding if they are 6–59 months old then you should only take this group from the whole population. Similarly, most feeding programmes admit children using percentage of the median. You should therefore calculate the number of children who are malnourished in the population, also using percentage of the median.

Example F2.2

Imagine there is an SFP for all moderately malnourished children aged 6–59 months and a TFP for severely malnourished children aged 6–59 months in District A. During the nutrition survey you estimate the prevalence of moderate malnutrition at 12% (95% CIs 9–15%) (<80% and >=70% median) and the prevalence of severe malnutrition at 3% (<70% median). The total population of the district is estimated at 123,000 people, of whom 17% are thought to be aged 6–59 months. In the previous week, 996 children under 5 years were registered in the SFP and 78 children under 5 years in the TFP. What are the programme's coverage rates, as estimated by the indirect method?

$$\text{SFP coverage} = 100 \times \frac{996}{0.12 \times (0.17 \times 123,000)}$$

$$= 39.7\%$$

$$\text{TFP coverage} = 100 \times \frac{78}{0.03 \times (0.17 \times 123,000)}$$

$$= 12.4\%$$

To calculate the sample size using the indirect method, the following calculations should be used:

Upper CI = $\dfrac{\text{number of children attending}}{\text{Lower CI of the estimated prevalence} \times \text{estimated number of children in population}} \times 100$

Lower CI = $\dfrac{\text{number of children attending}}{\text{Upper CI of the estimated prevalence} \times \text{estimated number of children in population}} \times 100$

Therefore, to calculate the CIs for the coverage of supplementary feeding calculated in Example F2.2 you would need to do the following calculation:

Upper CI = $\dfrac{996}{0.09 \times (0.17 \times 123,000)} \times 100 = 52.9\%$

Lower CI = $\dfrac{996}{0.15 \times (0.17 \times 123,000)} \times 100 = 31.8\%$

Therefore the estimation of coverage is 39.7% (31.8–52.9).

F2.2 Disadvantages of the standard methods

The standard methods of estimating programme coverage have two major problems. The first problem is connected to sample size and the second to the assumption of homogeneity.

F2.2.1 Sample size issues

The sample size calculated for an anthropometric survey allows the *prevalence* of acute malnutrition to be estimated with reasonable precision, but the sample size available to estimate *coverage* depends on the prevalence of acute malnutrition found by the survey. When the aim of the survey is to estimate the coverage of a feeding programme for *severe* acute malnutrition (a TFP), the sample size will usually be too small to estimate coverage with reasonable precision. This means that you will have very wide CIs around your estimate of coverage. This problem affects both direct and indirect methods of estimating coverage. This problem will be less acute if you are estimating the coverage of an SFP (rather than a TFP) because there will be more moderately malnourished children in the population.

The indirect method suffers from a further drawback because the denominator used in the formula is subject to considerable uncertainty. The population estimate is usually derived from census data. In complex emergency situations, certain factors may lead to census data not being accurate (eg, political manipulation, the absence of a functioning civil society, population displacement, and poor security).

F2.2.2 Homogeneity

Both the direct and indirect methods of measuring coverage assume that coverage of the feeding programmes is homogeneous across the whole survey area and therefore can only give you a whole-area estimate of coverage.[1] In a small geographical area, such as a refugee camp, this assumption may be true. However, over a wider area the assumption is often unlikely to be true, especially for some centre-based programmes because coverage will be greater for areas close to centres. Also, in the start-up phase some villages may not have information about the existence of centre-based facilities.

In general, anthropometric surveys which have been sampled using the two-stage cluster sample technique include more children from the most populous parts of the survey area (because a cluster is more likely to be sample from this area) than from the outlying areas. The most populous areas are more likely to have a feeding centre and hence the coverage of the programme is likely to be higher in these areas. Therefore, it is likely that the survey will overestimate coverage.

Both direct or indirect methods only produce one figure for the coverage of the whole survey area. If the homogeneity assumption is untrue and coverage is uneven then it is useful to be able to identify where coverage is good and where it is bad so you can improve your programme. The method described below is one way to do this.

F2.3 Centric systematic area sampling

The centric systematic area sampling (CSAS) method is a useful way to assess TFP coverage in an area where the coverage is not homogeneous and population figures are unsure (Myatt et al, 2004). The CSAS method adopts active case-finding. The project area is split into quadrants (squares of approximately equal area) and cases of severe malnutrition are sought. A simple count is made of cases enrolled in the programme, compared with cases not enrolled in the programme. This figure can be compiled for all the quadrants to give an overall project

---

[1] Note that the standard sampling methods described in Chapter B2 make the same assumption about the prevalence of malnutrition: it is assumed that the prevalence of malnutrition is the same throughout the survey area.

coverage figure, or used separately to estimate coverage in each area. As more cases can be seen using the CSAS method the CIs are much narrower than when you use the standard methods.

F2.3.1 How to conduct a CSAS coverage survey

Step 1 : Find a map
The first step in the CSAS coverage survey is to find a map of the programme area. Try to find a map showing the location of towns and villages; a map of 1:50,000 scale is ideal.

Step 2 : Draw a grid

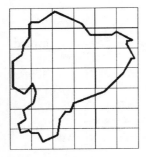

The next step is to draw a grid over the map. The size of each square should be small enough for it to be reasonable to assume that coverage will be similar throughout the square. A square of 10km by 10km will probably be small enough in most circumstances. Label each square with an x and y value – ie, starting with 1 on the bottom left corner going from left to right and starting with 1 in the bottom left corner going from bottom to top. This means that (in the diagram above) the square in the bottom left-hand corner has the co-ordinates 1,1. The square the bottom right has co-ordinates 6,1 and the square in the top right has co-ordinates 6,7.

Step 3 : Select the squares to sample
Select the squares with about 50% or more of their area inside the programme area.

Step 4 : Select the communities to sample
Select the community closest to the centre of each square. If the prevalence of malnutrition is low then you might need to select more than one community from each square. Determine the order in which communities should be sampled in advance of the fieldwork.

Step 5 : Case-finding

When you visit a community find cases using an active case-finding method. It is usually sufficient to ask community health workers, traditional birth attendants, traditional healers or other key informants to take you to see children who are sick, thin, or have swollen legs or feet. Then ask mothers of confirmed cases to help you find more. You could also use door-to-door screening. It is important that the case-finding method you use finds all, or nearly all, cases in the sampled communities. For each child measured and suspected of being a case, the carer should be asked whether the child is currently enrolled in the programme. Each case is confirmed by applying the programme's entry criteria (eg, age and < 70% WHM and/or bilateral pitting oedema). Remember to follow up children reported to be in a therapeutic feeding centre or at a distribution point on the day of the survey.

Step 6 : Record the data

Record the data on a form similar to that shown in Table F2.2. For each sampled community, you need to record the number of children in the programme (column 4), severely malnourished children in the programme (column 6), and the number of severely malnourished children (column 5). The population of the sampled communities can be a rough estimate based on roof counts or on information provided by reliable key informants. If this information is not available, every row in column 1 in Table F2.2 should be entered with 1.

At the end of your survey you should have filled in a form which will look something like the one shown in Table F2.2.

Step 7 : Calculate coverage

Two estimates of coverage can be calculated:

*   *point cover*, which counts only those people who on the day of the survey meet the eligibility criteria for the therapeutic feeding centre
*   *period cover*, which counts as cases those who exceed the eligibility criteria (perhaps because they are in the recovery phase).

The spreadsheet CSAScoverempty.xls, on the CD-ROM which accompanies this manual, allows you to enter the data, after which it will automatically calculate the coverage and plot the data on a map. CSAScoverexample.xls provides an example of a completed spreadsheet. The spreadsheets also provide an average of the coverage (either point or period cover) for the whole area, and it calculates CIs.

Table F2.2 Sample form for data collection in a coverage survey using the CSAS method

Population of the sampled communities	Quadrant reference (x)	Quadrant reference (y)	Number of children in the programme	Number of severely mal-nourished child-ren (cases)	Number of cases in the programme
456	4	1	4	7	2
567	4	2	3	4	0
123	4	3	1	4	1
345	4	4	1	3	1
362	4	5	3	3	1
233	4	6	1	5	1
346	4	7	1	3	0
186	4	8	1	2	0
246	4	9	0	3	0
outside survey area	4	10	–	–	–
123	5	1	3	5	2
234	5	2	4	2	0
256	5	3	1	4	1
270	5	4	0	5	0
175	5	5	4	5	2
138	5	6	2	8	1
268	5	7	1	6	0
301	5	8	1	6	1
	etc	..		..	..

Point cover is calculated as:

$$\frac{\text{number of cases in feeding programme}}{\text{total number of cases}} \times 100$$

Period cover is calculated as:

$$\frac{\text{number of children in feeding programme}}{\text{number of cases \textbf{not} in feeding programme} + \text{number of children in feeding programme}} \times 100$$

Step 8 : Plot the data

Coverage data is plotted as a mesh map and as a histogram. The level of black filling in the squares reflects the level of coverage found in each square (calculated in Step 7). For example, Table F2.2 shows that the quadrant with co-ordinates

(4,1) had seven cases, and two of them were enrolled in the programme. Figure F2.1 shows that the square 4 along from the left on the bottom of the diagram is approximately 1/3 filled with black to represent the extent of coverage in this area. The open squares indicate quadrants with zero coverage or quadrants where no communities have been sampled. You might find it helpful to mark the location of feeding centres, distribution points, health posts, roads and boundaries of the survey area on the map. This will help you interpret the results of the coverage survey.

Figure F2.1 Example of point coverage mesh map

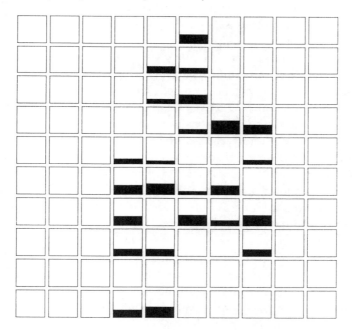

F2.3.2 Advantages of the CSAS method

The main advantage of the CSAS method is that you can see the spatial distribution of your programme's coverage. From the example above, you can see which communities are using the programme and which aren't. This is very useful because it means you can follow up on the communities in the quadrants which aren't using the programme and find out why.

Another major advantage of the CSAS method is that you can use it to refer children to the programme immediately. This, of course, is true of the direct method too – when you find a malnourished child who is not enrolled on a programme then you should always refer them if a programme is available. However, because the CSAS sees so many malnourished children (because of the active case-finding method) you are able to refer more of them than by using the direct or indirect survey methods.

F2.3.3 Potential disadvantages of the CSAS method

The CSAS method assumes that the coverage of a programme is homogeneous within any given quadrant. If the coverage is not homogeneous within each quadrant then the method will have the same problems as those described in Section F2.2. In fact, quadrants are normally relatively small areas – certainly much smaller than the whole programme area – so it is likely that the homogeneity assumption is true. If you are worried that the quadrants are not homogeneous, you could consider taking a greater number of smaller-sized quadrants for your survey.

A poor case-finding method might systematically exclude some children. For example, children from minority groups or children living on the periphery of sampled communities may be excluded, leading to bias. To avoid this you need to work really hard at your active case finding. Remind your key informants that you want to see all the sick or malnourished children in the community – not just the ones living in the centre of the village.

The method takes longer than the standard approaches because you spend one whole day in each quadrant, rather than just combining the coverage questions with a standard anthropometric survey. But also remember that active case finding is central to successful programme implementation. The estimation of the coverage can be integrated into programme outreach work. This would allow continued estimation of coverage as part of routine programme activity.

Finally, there is one important drawback of the method, which is this: although trials of CSAS methods indicate that very good results are obtained when estimating coverage of programmes designed to correct severe acute malnutrition (Myatt et al, 2004), results for SFPs (moderate malnutrition) are less accurate. This is because it is relatively straightforward for members of the community to identify severely malnourished children but harder for them to identify moderately malnourished children. This means that more moderately malnourished children will be missed by the active case-finding method and that the estimate of coverage for an SFP may be less accurate.

F2.4 What method of estimating coverage is most appropriate when?

All of the methods described above have some drawbacks. These are summarised in the Table F2.3. The Xs in the table show which method suffers from which drawback.

The most desirable method is the one which has the least drawbacks. Judging

Table F2.3 Summary of drawbacks faced by each of the coverage methods

Drawback	Method		
	Direct	**Indirect**	**CSAS**
Sample size too small	X	X	
Assumes homogeneity	X	X	
Cannot visualise distribution	X	X	
Need accurate population figures		X	
Less useful for active case finding	X	X	
Not useful for SFP			X
More time required			X

from this table, it looks as though the indirect method is the least useful, although it could be used to gain an interim estimate before a coverage survey could be conducted. In particular, the need for accurate population data means that in most situations this method will probably return inaccurate results. The exception to this rule may be in a camp situation where you are pretty sure of the population figures and that programme coverage is homogeneous.

From Table F2.3, it looks as though the CSAS method is the most promising, at least when you are trying to estimate the coverage of a TFP. The fact that the CSAS method can be incorporated into standard programme outreach activities gives it a big advantage over the other methods but means it may not easily be incorporated into a nutrition assessment. The CSAS method is particularly relevant in a setting where you suspect that the rates of coverage will differ substantially within the programme area. So it may be very useful to use it near the beginning of a programme – it will help you see where you need to work on improving coverage.

When you are estimating coverage of an SFP it may be necessary to use the direct method. The problems with sample size should not be so serious when you are estimating the coverage rate of an SFP (compared with a TFP) because you would expect to find more moderately malnourished children. However, the assumption about heterogeneity may still be a problem.

F2.5 Interpreting coverage data

The Sphere Project handbook (2004) suggests that coverage of both therapeutic and supplementary feeding programmes should be more than 50% in rural areas, more than 70% in urban areas and more than 90% in a camp setting.

Clearly, coverage can be affected by the acceptability of the programme, the location of the distribution points, the security situation (for staff and beneficiaries), the waiting time, the service quality and the extent of home visiting. If the coverage of your programme is lower than the criteria set by the Sphere guidelines then you need to investigate what the problem is.

Example F2.3

You estimate your TFP coverage in a survey at only 15%. You need to investigate why. Talk to the local authorities, local leaders, mothers and other carers. Is the TFP centre located in an appropriate area? Would a home-based treatment programme be more convenient for the population? Should you open another centre in the area? Do carers need assistance in travelling to the centre? Has the centre got a bad reputation for some reason? Is this bad reputation justified? How can you improve the situation? Do enough of the population know about the centre? Do you need to do more outreach work? Is another screening necessary? Etc.

Summary

- Programme coverage is an important indicator for monitoring and evaluating emergency nutrition interventions. Coverage data is also useful to help project staff find out how well a project is doing and whether or not it is meeting, or will meet, its objectives.
- The standard methods for collecting coverage data are not ideal because they assume that programme coverage is homogeneous throughout the survey area and only provide a single-area estimate. The direct method is probably the best method for assessing coverage of supplementary feeding programmes.
- The centric systematic area sampling (CSAS) method can be a useful way to assess therapeutic feeding programme coverage in an area where the coverage is not homogeneous. The project area is split into quadrants (squares of approximately equal area) and cases of severe malnutrition are sought actively.
- If selective feeding programmes have coverage rates of less than 50% in rural areas, 70% in urban areas and 90% in camp areas, it is important to find out why the coverage is low.

Annex S1
List of useful websites for secondary information

Previous nutrition surveys and young child feeding information

Unicef statistical data by country
http://www.unicef.org/statis

Health Information Network for Advanced Planning
http://www.hinap.org/

WHO Global database on child growth and malnutrition
http://www.who.int/nutgrowthdb/

MACRO International Demographic and Health Surveys
http://www.macroint.com/dhs/

Results from multi-indicator cluster surveys
http://www.childinfo.org/

Nutrition-related data for Africa
http://www.africanutrition.net/

Nutrition in crisis situations (formerly the Refugee Nutrition Information System) is published every three months
http://www.unsystem.org/scn/Publications/html/rnis.html

Food security reports

Save the Children UK
www.savethechildren.org.uk/foodsecurity/documentation/index.htm

> Baselines, national and local household economy reports, some nutrition surveys. Organised by region.

FEWS-Net
www.fews.net

> 'Livelihoods' section includes baseline reports and some Livelihood Zones maps and explanations under 'resources'

'Hazards' and 'Risk Analysis' sections have some food economy reports in different sub-sections, particularly under 'Special Reports'

WFP Vulnerability Analysis & Mapping (VAM)
www.wfp.org

Follow links to Operations – VAM – VAM by Country *and* VAM Library for assessment reports and secondary resources

FAO – Global Information and Early Warning System (GIEWS)
www.fao.org/giews

Reports predominantly on crop/agricultural situation by country. 'Special Reports' section includes FAO/ WFP Crop and Food Supply Assessment Mission reports which include sections on vulnerability.

General information on emergencies

Reliefweb
http://www.reliefweb.int/w/rwb.nsf
information for the humanitarian community on emergencies, including situation reports and maps.

Global IDP Project
http://www.idpproject.org
Reports on the situations of IDPs worldwide

Integrated Regional Information Network (IRIN)
http://www.irinnews.org
Situation reports and up to date information on emergencies.

Appendix S2
Anthropometric measurement of children aged 6–59 months

S1.1 Specifications for weighing and measuring equipment

A brief description of the specifications of weighing and measurement equipment suitable for anthropometric surveys is given in table S1.1.

S2.1.1 Weighing equipment

A suitable instrument for weighing children aged 6–59 months is a 25kg hanging spring scale marked out in steps of 0.1kg. Weighing pants should be provided with the scale. Normally, Salter scales are used. Salter scales can sometimes be bought in a country, although they may be of poor quality. Most country programmes order the scales from overseas or from Unicef.

S2.1.2 Equipment for measuring height and length

A measuring board is normally at least 130cm long, is made of hardwood and has a hard water-resistant finish. The board should have a metal tape-measure attached to it, which should be marked out in 0.1cm steps.[1] The head board must be movable and the foot board must be large enough for a child to stand on it.

Height boards are usually ordered from carpenters, although you may obtain them from Save the Children head office, or from Unicef in some cases.

A height arch can be used for selecting children shorter than 110cm. This can be constructed simply and should consist of a horizontal bar fixed at 110cm above the ground at right angles to a vertical pole (or between two vertical poles). Any child who can walk under this horizontal bar without hitting it, and without stooping, should be included in the sample for further measuring.

---

[1] Note that metal can get very hot in the sun so keep equipment in the shade.

Table S2.1 Recommended measuring equipment

Name of product	Salter hanging scale	Seca 835	Wooden height boards. As supplied in nutrition kits	Leicester height measure	TALC MUAC tapes
Price in January 2004	£50	£185	£18.40	£58	£0.28 each
Maximum / minimum	0–25kg	0–136kg	0–130cm	75–205cm	0–390mm
Gradations	100g	20g for babies 100g for adults	1mm	1mm	1mm
Other details	Robust, reliable suspended weighing scale provided with weighing pants	Combined adult/baby digital scale (using batteries) which has a removable baby tray, weight hold, tare and power down features.	Wooden height/ length board + head block	This measure is used by Unicef and is lightweight. Consists of a foot plate with a 4-section measuring column. Complete with lightweight, portable case.	Durable material
Recommended use	Nutrition surveys for children under five years of age	Nutrition surveys including infants <6 months and older children and adults. TFCs	Nutrition surveys 6–59 months	Nutrition surveys of adults. TFCs admitting adults	Nutrition surveys to complement WFH. Two-stage screening.

S2.1.3 Equipment for measuring mid-upper arm circumference

Mid-upper arm circumference (MUAC) measurements should be made using a flexible, non-stretch tape made of fibreglass. Alternatively a fibreglass insertion tape can be used.

Some agencies (such as Oxfam and Action Contre la Faim – ACF) have produced specially made MUAC tapes for use in nutrition screenings. These are colour banded so that the measurer knows whether or not to refer a child for further (weight and height) measurements. You can also get MUAC tapes from TALC (see Table S2.1).

S2.2 Measuring children aged 6–59 months

S2.2.1 Estimating age

Emergency nutrition surveys normally measure the weight and height of children aged 6–59 months. However, in many rural areas of the developing world, the age of children is not known. In general, the younger the child is, the more accurately you can estimate her/his month of birth.

The following methods are helpful for determining or estimating the age of a child, if the mother does not know.

- Look up age in official registers. In rural communities, you normally cannot find local official registers of births or a baptismal certificate book. Instead, some households may have the child's immunisation card. If health workers properly recorded the date of birth on the immunisation card, then you can copy the date from the card. Therefore, when trying to determine a child's age, you should always ask to see the child's immunisation card.
- Use the birth date of a neighbour's child as a reference. If the age of a neighbour's child is known, then you can ask other women whether or not their child was born before or after the reference child.
- Use a local events calendar. A local events calendar shows all the dates on which important events took place during the past five years. It can show local holidays, hailstorms, the opening of a nearby school or clinic and political elections, etc. An example of a local events calendar (designed for Gubalafto Woreda in North Wollo, Ethiopia) is given in Table S1.2. You should ask the mother whether or not the child was born before or after a certain event, and work out a fairly accurate age in this way.

Estimating age from height

The World Health Organization (WHO) recommends that if, for some reason, no age data are available and a local events calendar cannot be used to estimate

Table S2.2 Example of a local events calendar from Ethiopia to estimate age in children aged 6–59 months for a survey conducted in November 1994. Ages shown are months.

Month	1989–90	age	1990–91	age	1991–92	age	1992–93	age	1993–94	age		1994–95 age
September	New year Meskel	62	New Year Meskel	50	New Year Meskel	38	New Year Meskel	26	New Year Meskel	14	New Year Meskel	2
October	Green cereals Ramadan	61	Green cereals	49	Green cereals	37	Green cereals	25	Green cereals	13	Green cereals	1
November	Meher	60	Meher Ramadan	48	Meher Ramadan	36	Meher	24	Meher	12		
December	Christmas	59	Christmas	47	Christmas	35	Christmas Ramadan	23	Christmas Ramadan	11		
January	Epiphany Arafat	58	Epiphany Arafat	46	Epiphany	34	Epiphany	22	Epiphany	10		
February		57	Arafat	45	Arafat	33	Arafat	21	Arafat	9		
March		56		44		32		20		8		
April	Good Friday Easter	55	Good Friday Easter	43	Good Friday Easter	31	Good Friday Easter	19	Good Friday Easter	7		
May	Mewlid	54	Mewlid	42		30		18		6		
June	Belg harvest	53	Mewlid Belg harvest	41	Mewlid Belg harvest	29	Mewlid Belg harvest	17	Mewlid Belg harvest	5		
July	Kremt rain	52	Kremt rain	40	Kremt rain	28	Kremt rain	16	Kremt rain	4		
August	Weeding	51	Weeding	39	Weeding	27	Weeding	15	Weeding	3		

the age of the children, then it may be useful to use a height cut-off instead.

- Originally, WHO recommended measuring children between 65cm and 110cm, as an equivalent to children aged 6–59 months. These heights were chosen because 65cm is the length median in the National Centre for Health Statistics (NCHS) reference of children aged six months and 110cm is the height median for children aged 60 months.
- More recently, WHO has recommended that only children 65–100cm tall should be included in nutrition surveys for children aged 6–59 months, in countries where the prevalence of stunting is known to be high (WHO, 2000).

In fact, both of these recommendations are likely to lead to a bias in the estimate of malnutrition if the population is stunted. Consider the two options:

- The height cut-off is fixed at 110 cm, but the population is stunted and the mean height of children aged 60 months is 100cm. Then the sample will:
  - include children older than 59 months
  - include a disproportionate number of stunted children.

- The height cut-off is fixed at 100cm, which is the same as the mean height of children aged 60 months. Then the sample will:
  - exclude older children of normal height (eg, age 58 months)
  - exclude younger, taller children (eg, age 54 months).

Older children are less likely to be wasted, but stunted children are more likely to be wasted. Thus, both of the recommendations will be biased towards older, stunted children.

Save the Children UK has recently completed an analysis of 66 survey datasets to review the effect of excluding taller children. The analysis found that, in fact, the prevalence of acute malnutrition defined in z-scores did not change significantly when the height range was changed. However, the prevalence of acute malnutrition defined in terms of WHMs was lowered when the taller children were excluded (ie, height cut-off of 100cm).

Because of these problems in using height as a proxy for age it is strongly recommended that you use a local events calendar to ascertain the age of children in an emergency nutrition assessment. However, if this is not possible then we recommend using the 65–110cm cut-off until further research has validated another method.[2] This means that if the child is under 5 years but more than 110cm they should be included in the survey.

---

[2] We make this recommendation because future surveys will then be directly comparable to earlier surveys.

S2.2.2 Weight

Weight should be measured to the nearest 100g. Although various types of scales are used for weighing young children in the field, the most commonly used is the hanging spring balance, which can weigh up to 25kg. Hanging scales are robust, cheap and easy to carry.

Calibration of the scales should be checked immediately before, and during, each session (eg, at the start of each cluster), using the same known weights. The scales should first be set at zero, with the weighing pants or basket attached. Suitable items for the calibration include a stone or a standard 5–10kg weight. Spring balance scales should be replaced whenever the springs are so stretched that readings are incorrect.

Figure S2.1 shows the correct procedure for weighing a child with a hanging spring balance. Additional notes are provided below:

1. Explain the procedure to the child's mother or carer before starting.
2. Install a 25kg hanging spring scale (graduated by 100g). If mobile weighing is needed, the scale can be hooked on a tree or a stick held by two people.
3. Suspend weighing pants from the lower hook of the scale and recalibrate to zero.
4. Remove the child's clothes, and any jewellery and place her/him in the weighing pants (older children may hold on to the bar and lift themselves off the ground).
5. Ensure nothing is touching the child.
6. Read the scale at eye level (if the child is moving about and the needle does not stabilise, estimate weight by using the value situated at the midpoint of the range of oscillations).
7. Announce the value to the assistant, who repeats, verifies and records.

In cold climates it may not be appropriate or acceptable to weigh children without their clothes on. In this situation careful preparation before the survey should be conducted so that children can be weighed already clothed. This involves preparing:

- a reference sheet of the weights and descriptions of popular children's clothing items based on the child's age and the season in which the survey is being conducted
- an album with photographs of different items of clothing with a description of the item, its principle fabric, the age of the children wearing it and its weight.

The team needs to be carefully trained to recognise the items accurately. In the analysis, the weight of each child's clothing should be subtracted from the weight

Figure S2.1 How to take weight of a child using hanging scales*

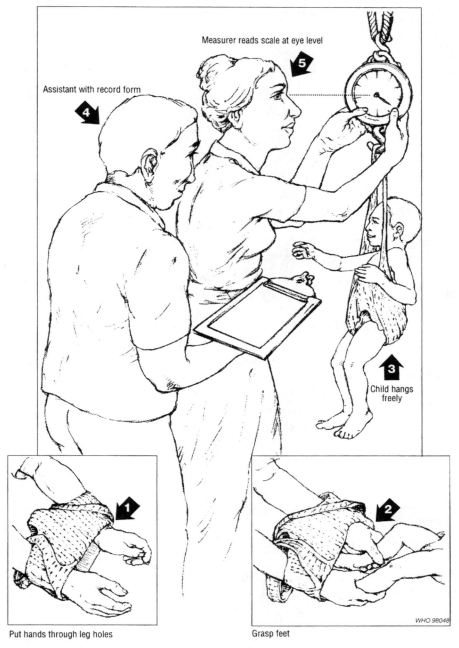

Measurer reads scale at eye level

Assistant with record form

Child hangs freely

Put hands through leg holes

Grasp feet

WHO 98048

* Adapted, with permission, from *Assessing the nutritional status of young children* (preliminary version). New York, United Nations Department of Technical Co-operation for Development and Statistical Office, 1990.

measured. This can result in an accurate estimate of the child's weight. More information on how to do this can be found in Tuan et al (2002).

S2.2.3 Height and length

Every effort should be made to measure children's height accurately, to the nearest 0.1cm if possible. Measurement errors of 2–3cm can easily occur and cause significant errors in classifying nutrition status.

Children less than 24 months of age (or up to 85cm in height) are measured supine (lying down) on a horizontal measuring board. Children aged 24–59 months (or above 85cm) should be measured standing up (WHO, 2000).

Once a child can stand it is easier and more convenient to measure her/him standing up – children are also normally happier to stand than to lie down (it is less frightening for them). In terms of accuracy, it is important to follow the rule that children must be measured in a lying position when they are younger than 24 months and in a standing position when they are older than 23 months. This is because this was how the NCHS/Centers for Disease Control and Prevention (CDC)/WHO reference children were measured, and individuals measured in the lying position are taller (on average between 0.5 and 1.5cm) than individuals measured in the standing position. Thus, if you measure children in a different way from that used to measure the children in the reference tables, you have to adjust for this when you are comparing their heights.[3]

Figure S1.2 shows the correct procedure for measuring the length of a child less than 24 months. Additional notes are provided below:

1. Explain the procedure to the child's mother or carer.
2. Remove the child's shoes and any hair ornament or top knot on the child's head.
3. Place the child gently on to the board, with the head against the fixed vertical part, and the soles of the feet near the cursor or moving part. The child should lie straight in the middle of the board, looking directly up.
4. The assistant should hold the child's head firmly against the base of the board, while the measurer places one hand on the knees (to keep the legs straight) and places the child's feet flat against the cursor with the other hand.
5. The measurer reads and announces the length to the nearest 0.1cm.
6. The assistant repeats and verifies the measurement and then records it.

---

[3] In some programmes all children are measured lying down. This is not recommended. However, if you are analysing this type of data you need to calculate the height of the older children ≥ 85cm) by taking 1cm off the recorded length measure.

Figure S2.2 How to measure length of a child <24 months

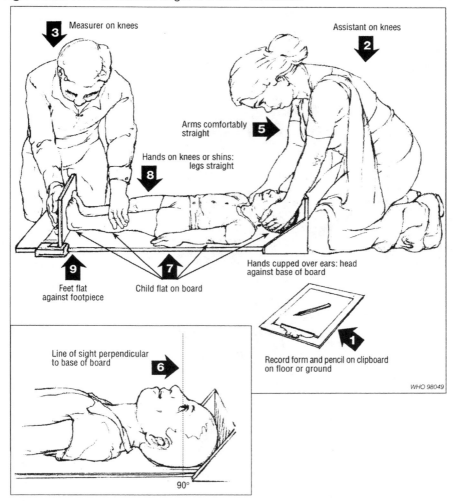

Measurer on knees

Assistant on knees

Arms comfortably straight

Hands on knees or shins: legs straight

Hands cupped over ears: head against base of board

Feet flat against footpiece

Child flat on board

Line of sight perpendicular to base of board

Record form and pencil on clipboard on floor or ground

WHO 98049

90°

* Adapted, with permission, from *Assessing the nutritional status of young children* (preliminary version). New York, United Nations Department of Technical Co-operation for Development and Statistical Office, 1990.

Note: In some cultures, measuring a child lying down is related to death (measurement of the coffin). Where this occurs, information and education sessions may be held to prepare the mothers for this kind of procedure.

Figure S2.3 shows the correct procedure for measuring the height of a child more than 24 months. Additional notes are provided below:

1. Explain the procedure to the child's mother or carer.

Figure S2.3 How to measure height in a child ≥ 24 months

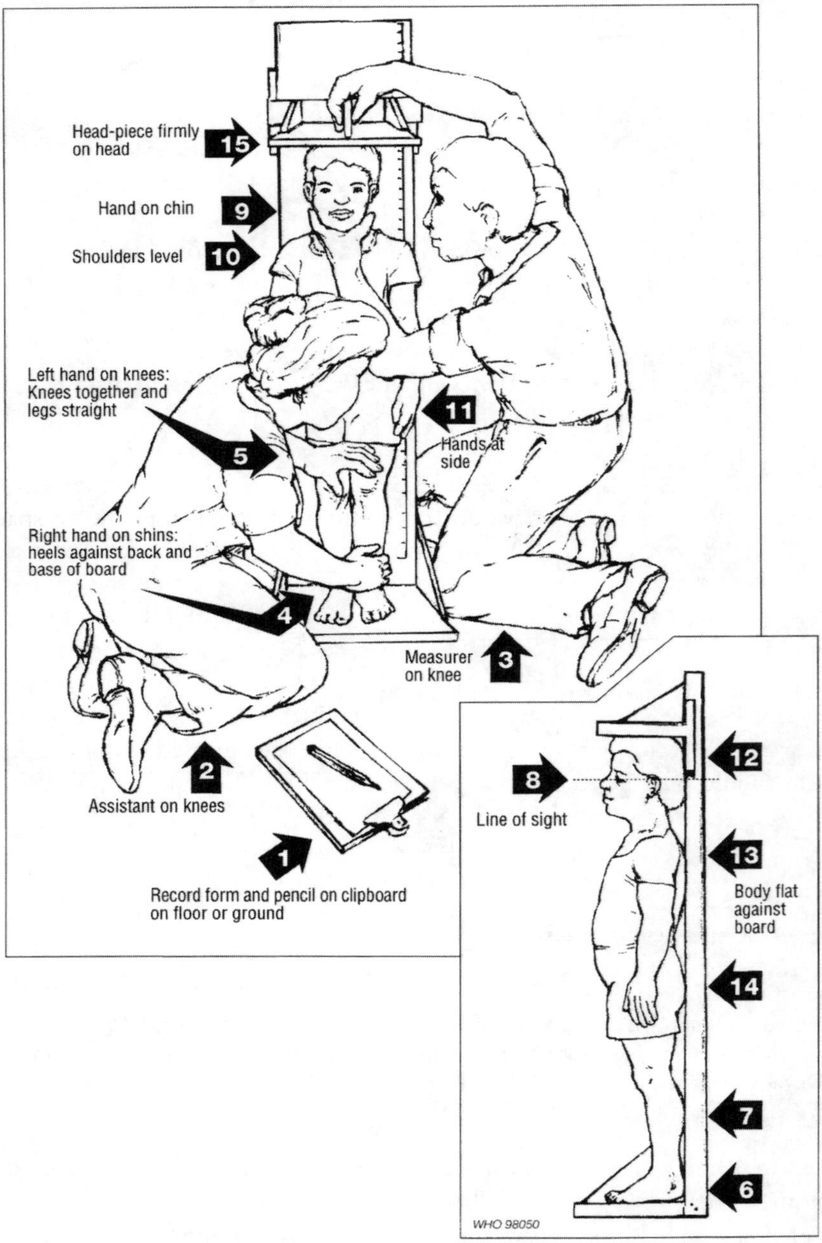

Head-piece firmly on head **15**

Hand on chin **9**

Shoulders level **10**

Left hand on knees: Knees together and legs straight **5**

11 Hands at side

Right hand on shins: heels against back and base of board **4**

Measurer on knee **3**

2 Assistant on knees

1 Record form and pencil on clipboard on floor or ground

8 Line of sight

12

13 Body flat against board

14

7

6

WHO 98050

* Adapted, with permission, from *Assessing the nutritional status of young children* (preliminary version). New York, United Nations Department of Technical Co-operation for Development and Statistical Office, 1990.

2. Place the measuring board upright in a location where there is room for movement around the board.
3. Remove the child's shoes and any hair ornament or top knot on the child's head and stand her/him on the middle of the measuring board.
4. An assistant should firmly press the child's ankles and knees against the board.
5. Ensure that the child's head, shoulders, buttocks, knees and heels touch the board.
6. The measurer should position the head and the cursor at right angles – the mid-ear and eye socket should be in line and hair should be compressed by the cursor.
7. The measurer reads and announces the height to the nearest 0.1cm.
8. The assistant repeats and verifies the measurement and then records it.

S2.2.4 Oedema

Oedema is the retention of water and sodium in the extra-cellular spaces. Generally it accounts for 10–30% of bodyweight, but in the most severe cases of kwashiorkor the proportion can reach 50%. To diagnose oedema, moderate thumb pressure is applied to just above the ankle or the tops of the feet for about three seconds (if you count 'one thousand and one, one thousand and two, one thousand and three' in English, pronouncing the words carefully, this takes about three seconds). If there is oedema, an impression remains for some time (at least a few seconds) where the oedema fluid has been pressed out of the tissue. A child should only be recorded as oedematous if both feet have oedema.

Figure S2.4 shows how to check for oedema.

Figure S2.4 How to check for oedema

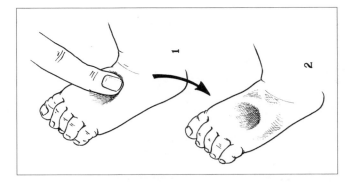

Figure S2.5 How to measure MUAC*

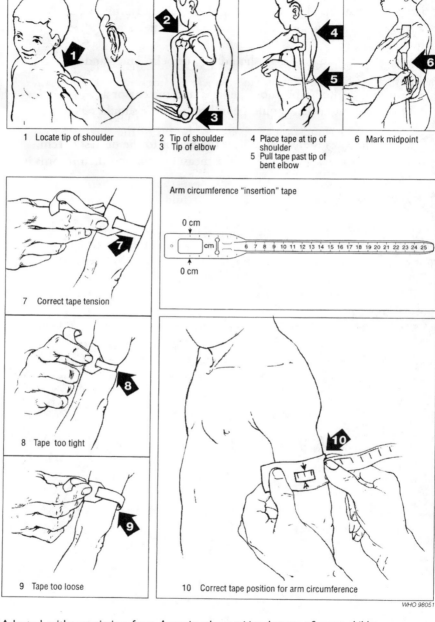

1   Locate tip of shoulder

2   Tip of shoulder
3   Tip of elbow

4   Place tape at tip of shoulder
5   Pull tape past tip of bent elbow

6   Mark midpoint

7   Correct tape tension

Arm circumference "insertion" tape

0 cm

0 cm

8   Tape too tight

9   Tape too loose

10   Correct tape position for arm circumference

WHO 98051

*Adapted, with permission, from *Assessing the nutritional status of young children* (preliminary version). New York, United Nations Department of Technical Co-operation for Development and Statistical Office, 1990.

S1.2.6 MUAC

Arm circumference is measured on the upper left arm. Measurements should be made to the nearest millimetre.

Figure S2.5 shows the correct procedure for measuring the MUAC of a child. Additional notes are provided below:

1. Explain the procedure to the child's mother or carer.
2. If possible, the child should stand erect and sideways to the measurer.
3. Bend the left arm at 90 degrees to the body.
4. Place a measuring tape along the upper arm and find the mid-point of the upper arm. The mid-point is between the tip of the shoulder (olecranon) and the elbow (acromion process).
5. Mark the mid-upper arm point with a pen.
6. Let the left arm hang relaxed at the side of the body.
7. Place the MUAC measuring tape on the midway point.
8. Pull the tape until it fits securely around the arm. The tape should not be left too slack nor pulled too tightly. The tape should touch the skin all the way around the arm, but not make a dent in the skin.
9. Read the measurement at the window of the tape measure.
10. Record mid-arm circumference to the nearest 0.1cm.

Note: MUAC measurement is fast and simple, but not easy, and variations in measurements often occur between different measurers. This is mainly related to how the tape is pulled or squeezed around the arm.

S2.3 Height-for-age cut-off points

The following cut-off points are commonly used to classify chronic malnutrition, or stunting.

Table S2.3 Height-for-age cut-off points in children aged 6–59 months

Category	Percentage of the median	z-scores
Severe	< 80 %	< −3 z-scores
Moderate	< 90% to > = 80%	< −2 z-scores to > = −3 z-scores
Global	< 90%	< −2 z-scores

S2.4 Weight-for-age cut-off points

Table S1.4 Weight-for-age cut-off points in children aged 6–59 months (Cogill, 2003)

System	Cut-off	Malnutrition classification
WHO	< −1 to ≥ −2 z-score	mild
	< −2 to ≥ −3 z-score	moderate
	< −3 z-score	severe
Road-to-Health charts	≥ 80% of median	normal
	≥ 60% − < 80% of median	mild-to-moderate
	< 60% of median	severe
Gomez classification	≥ 90% of median	normal
	≥ 75% − < 90% of median	mild
	≥ 60% − < 75% of median	moderate
	< 60% of median	severe

Appendix S3
How to standardise measurements among team members

The training of personnel to make and record specific measurements includes not only theoretical explanations and demonstrations, but also an opportunity for participants to practise the measurement techniques, as well as reading and recording the results. Once all trainees have adequately practised the measurement and recording techniques, and feel comfortable with their performance, standardisation exercises can be carried out.

The standardisation test consists of repeating a measure twice on 10 different children, with a time interval between measures on the same child. The size of the variation between repeated measures is calculated to assess precision, and the mean measure is calculated to assess accuracy. Each enumerator is then given a score of competence in performing measures. Any misunderstandings and/or measuring errors can then be corrected during the training process.

Definitions of accuracy and precision are given below:

- Accuracy: ability to obtain a measurement that will duplicate as closely as possible to the real value.
- Precision: ability to repeat a measurement on the same subject with a minimum variation.

These two abilities are complementary. An enumerator may be precise but not accurate: he finds a wrong value for the measure, but he 'precisely' finds the same wrong value every time. In the same way, an enumerator may be accurate but not precise, meaning the mean measure on a number of measures is close to the real measure, but wide variation between measures exists.

S3.1 Practical organisation of the test

The exercise is performed with a group of ten children whose ages fall within the pre-established range for the study (normally 6–59 months). Each child which will be measured should also be given an ID starting from 1. Before carrying out the standardisation exercise, the supervisor carefully weighs and measures each child and records the results without any of the trainees seeing the results. The supervisor is automatically given the ID number 0. The supervisor should start by filling in a form like that shown in Figure S3.1.

Figure: S3.1 Sample format for the supervisor (length and height measurements shown)

| Child | Supervisor | |
No	1st measure	2nd measure
1	828	822
2	838	846
3	860	856
4	862	860
5	820	820
6	856	854
7	823	824
8	876	876
9	801	806
10	853	865

Each trainee (known as an evaluator) should also be given an ID starting from 1. So if you have 6 trainees they should be numbered 1–6.

For each exercise, a group of trainees will conduct the measurements in a pre-determined order. Each child will remain at a fixed location with the ID number clearly marked by them. The distance between each child should be big enough to prevent the trainees seeing or hearing each other's results. You should decide whether you want to concentrate on weight, height or MUAC in the exercise (the exercise should be repeated for each type of measurement). Make it clear to the evaluators how the results should be recorded: ie, weight to the nearest 0.1kg, height to the nearest 0.1cm and MUAC in mm.

At the beginning of an exercise, position a pair of trainee measurers with each child. Then the supervisor should instruct the measurers to begin the measurements. The trainees should carefully conduct the measurements and clearly record the results on the second and third columns of the anthropometric standardisation form (see Figure S3.2) next to the child's identification number. Each pair of measurers should have their own form to complete and each should have turn at taking the measurement. When each member of the pair has done the measurement they should move on to the next child. At the end the whole process should be repeated so that each enumerator has two measures for each child.

Use the same equipment to measure each child's weight and height. Trainee measurers and assistant should rotate to conduct the measurement, but the equipment remains stationed next to each child. Only one pair of measurers should be with a child at any one time. Talking between pairs of trainee measurers during this exercise should not be allowed.

Figure S3.2 Sample format for the enumerators (height measurements shown)

Child No	Enumerator 1	
	1st measure	2nd measure
1	842	837
2	861	854
3	862	858
4	875	865
5	826	827
6	864	860
7	820	835
8	884	882
9	820	815
10	866	870

The supervisor should take advantage of the standardisation exercises to observe systematically each trainee's performance. Observations should include checking their positioning of the equipment, adjustment to zero, positioning of child, child's clothing and angle at which the reading is taken, etc. If necessary, the supervisor should make notes on any errors to discuss with the team later.

S3.2 Analysis of the results of the test using SigmaD

SigmaD.exe is software designed to analyse the results from standardisation tests and determine how precise and accurate your enumerators are. The programme can be found in the CD-ROM attached to this manual. SigmaD has a very comprehensive help file attached to it.

You should install the software and start it. You will be asked whether you want to Create a new project or Open an existing project. To start with you should Create a new project. You will then be prompted to give the project a name. You will then need to enter the number of evaluators on your team (this is the same as trainees) and the number of subjects (ie, children who are being measured). You will then have a screen which allows you to enter the results from Figures S3.1 and S3.2 above. The first page is for the supervisors results and the subsequent pages for each enumerator (click on the tabs at the top of the screen).

When you have finished entering the data click on Report. You will then see starting from page 3 the results of each enumerator and a grade of how precise and how accurate each enumerator was. Those who graded Poor should be retrained and checked again.

Appendix S4
NCHS/CDC/WHO reference tables

Table S4.1 NCHS/CDC/WHO normalised reference weight for length/height (49–115 cm) by sex

Length/ height (cm)	Boys' weight (kg)				Girls' weight (kg)			
	Median	−1 SD	−2 SD	−3 SD	Median	−1 SD	−2 SD	−3 SD
49	3.1	2.8	2.5	2.1	3.3	2.9	2.6	2.2
49.5	3.2	2.9	2.5	2.1	3.4	3.0	2.6	2.2
50	3.3	2.9	2.5	2.2	3.4	3.0	2.6	2.3
50.5	3.4	3.0	2.6	2.2	3.5	3.1	2.7	2.3
51	3.5	3.1	2.6	2.2	3.5	3.1	2.7	2.3
51.5	3.6	3.1	2.7	2.3	3.6	3.2	2.8	2.4
52	3.7	3.2	2.8	2.3	3.7	3.3	2.8	2.4
52.5	3.8	3.3	2.8	2.4	3.8	3.4	2.9	2.5
53	3.9	3.4	2.9	2.4	3.9	3.4	3.0	2.5
53.5	4.0	3.5	3.0	2.5	4.0	3.5	3.1	2.6
54	4.1	3.6	3.1	2.6	4.1	3.6	3.1	2.7
54.5	4.2	3.7	3.2	2.6	4.2	3.7	3.2	2.7
55	4.3	3.8	3.3	2.7	4.3	3.8	3.3	2.8
55.5	4.5	3.9	3.3	2.8	4.4	3.9	3.4	2.9
56	4.6	4.0	3.5	2.9	4.5	4.0	3.5	3.0
56.5	4.7	4.1	3.6	3.0	4.6	4.1	3.6	3.0
57	4.8	4.3	3.7	3.1	4.8	4.2	3.7	3.1
57.5	5.0	4.4	3.8	3.2	4.9	4.3	3.8	3.2
58	5.1	4.5	3.9	3.3	5.0	4.4	3.9	3.3
58.5	5.2	4.6	4.0	3.4	5.1	4.6	4.0	3.4
59	5.4	4.8	4.1	3.5	5.3	4.7	4.1	3.5
59.5	5.5	4.9	4.2	3.6	5.4	4.8	4.2	3.6
60	5.7	5.0	4.4	3.7	5.5	4.9	4.3	3.7
60.5	5.8	5.1	4.5	3.8	5.7	5.1	4.4	3.8
61	5.9	5.3	4.6	4.0	5.8	5.2	4.6	3.9
61.5	6.1	5.4	4.8	4.1	6.0	5.3	4.7	4.0
62	6.2	5.6	4.9	4.2	6.1	5.4	4.8	4.1
62.5	6.4	5.7	5.0	4.3	6.2	5.6	4.9	4.2
63	6.5	5.8	5.2	4.5	6.4	5.7	5.0	4.4
63.5	6.7	6.0	5.3	4.6	6.5	5.8	5.2	4.5
64	6.8	6.1	5.4	4.7	6.7	6.0	5.3	4.6
64.5	7.0	6.3	5.6	4.9	6.8	6.1	5.4	4.7
65	7.1	6.4	5.7	5.0	7.0	6.3	5.5	4.8
65.5	7.3	6.5	5.8	5.1	7.1	6.4	5.7	4.9
66	7.4	6.7	6.0	5.3	7.3	6.5	5.8	5.1

Length/ height (cm)	Boys' weight (kg)				Girls' weight (kg)			
	Median	−1 SD	−2 SD	−3 SD	Median	−1 SD	−2 SD	−3 SD
66.5	7.6	6.8	6.1	5.4	7.4	6.7	5.9	5.2
67	7.7	7.0	6.2	5.5	7.5	6.8	6.0	5.3
67.5	7.8	7.1	6.4	5.7	7.7	6.9	6.2	5.4
68	8.0	7.3	6.5	5.8	7.8	7.1	6.3	5.5
68.5	8.1	7.4	6.6	5.9	8.0	7.2	6.4	5.6
69	8.3	7.5	6.8	6.0	8.1	7.3	6.5	5.8
69.5	8.4	7.7	6.9	6.2	8.2	7.5	6.7	5.9
70	8.5	7.8	7.0	6.3	8.4	7.6	6.8	6.0
70.5	8.7	7.9	7.2	6.4	8.5	7.7	6.9	6.1
71	8.8	8.1	7.3	6.5	8.6	7.8	7.0	6.2
71.5	8.9	8.2	7.4	6.7	8.8	8.0	7.1	6.3
72	9.1	8.3	7.5	6.8	8.9	8.1	7.2	6.4
72.5	9.2	8.4	7.7	6.9	9.0	8.2	7.4	6.5
73	9.3	8.6	7.8	7.0	9.1	8.3	7.5	6.6
73.5	9.5	8.7	7.9	7.1	9.3	8.4	7.6	6.7
74	9.6	8.8	8.0	7.2	9.4	8.5	7.7	6.8
74.5	9.7	8.9	8.1	7.3	9.5	8.6	7.8	6.9
75	9.8	9.0	8.2	7.4	9.6	8.7	7.9	7.0
75.5	9.9	9.1	8.3	7.5	9.7	8.8	8.0	7.1
76	10.0	9.2	8.4	7.6	9.8	8.9	8.1	7.2
76.5	10.2	9.3	8.5	7.7	9.9	9.0	8.2	7.3
77	10.3	9.4	8.6	7.8	10.0	9.1	8.3	7.4
77.5	10.4	9.5	8.7	7.9	10.1	9.2	8.4	7.5
78	10.5	9.7	8.8	8.0	10.2	9.3	8.5	7.6
78.5	10.6	9.8	8.9	8.1	10.3	9.4	8.6	7.7
79	10.7	9.9	9.0	8.2	10.4	9.5	8.7	7.8
79.5	10.8	10.0	9.1	8.2	10.5	9.6	8.7	7.9
80	10.9	10.1	9.2	8.3	10.6	9.7	8.8	8.0
80.5	11.0	10.1	9.3	8.4	10.7	9.8	8.9	8.0
81	11.1	10.2	9.4	8.5	10.8	9.9	9.0	8.1
81.5	11.2	10.3	9.5	8.6	10.9	10.0	9.1	8.2
82	11.3	10.4	9.6	8.7	11.0	10.1	9.2	8.3
82.5	11.4	10.5	9.6	8.8	11.1	10.2	9.3	8.4
83	11.5	10.6	9.7	8.8	11.2	10.3	9.4	8.5
83.5	11.6	10.7	9.8	8.9	11.3	10.4	9.5	8.6
84	11.7	10.8	9.9	9.0	11.4	10.5	9.6	8.7
84.5	11.8	10.9	10.0	9.1	11.5	10.6	9.6	8.7
85	12.1	11.0	9.9	8.9	11.8	10.8	9.7	8.6
85.5	12.2	11.1	10.0	8.9	11.9	10.9	9.8	8.7
86	12.3	11.2	10.1	9.0	12.0	11.0	9.9	8.8
86.5	12.5	11.3	10.2	9.1	12.2	11.1	10.0	8.9
87	12.6	11.5	10.3	9.2	12.3	11.2	10.1	9.0
87.5	12.7	11.6	10.4	9.3	12.4	11.3	10.2	9.1
88	12.8	11.7	10.5	9.4	12.5	11.4	10.3	9.2
88.5	12.9	11.8	10.6	9.5	12.6	11.5	10.4	9.3
89	13.0	11.9	10.7	9.6	12.7	11.6	10.5	9.3

Length/ height (cm)	Boys' weight (kg)				Girls' weight (kg)			
	Median	–1 SD	–2 SD	–3 SD	Median	–1 SD	–2 SD	–3 SD
89.5	13.1	12.0	10.8	9.7	12.8	11.7	10.6	9.4
90	13.3	12.1	10.9	9.8	12.9	11.8	10.7	9.5
90.5	13.4	12.2	11.0	9.9	13.0	11.9	10.7	9.6
91	13.5	12.3	11.1	9.9	13.2	12.0	10.8	9.7
91.5	13.6	12.4	11.2	10.0	13.3	12.1	10.9	9.8
92	13.7	12.5	11.3	10.1	13.4	12.2	11.0	9.9
92.5	13.9	12.6	11.4	10.2	13.5	12.3	11.1	9.9
93	14.0	12.8	11.5	10.3	13.6	12.4	11.2	10.0
93.5	14.1	12.9	11.6	10.4	13.7	12.5	11.3	10.1
94	14.2	13.0	11.7	10.5	13.9	12.6	11.4	10.2
94.5	14.3	13.1	11.8	10.6	14.0	12.8	11.5	10.3
95	14.5	13.2	11.9	10.7	14.1	12.9	11.6	10.4
95.5	14.6	13.3	12.0	10.8	14.2	13.0	11.7	10.5
96	14.7	13.4	12.1	10.9	14.3	13.1	11.8	10.6
96.5	14.8	13.5	12.2	11.0	14.5	13.2	11.9	10.7
97	15.0	13.7	12.4	11.0	14.6	13.3	12.0	10.7
97.5	15.1	13.8	12.5	11.1	14.7	13.4	12.1	10.8
98	15.2	13.9	12.6	11.2	14.9	13.5	12.2	10.9
98.5	15.4	14.0	12.7	11.3	15.0	13.7	12.3	11.0
99	15.5	14.1	12.8	11.4	15.1	13.8	12.4	11.1
99.5	15.6	14.3	12.9	11.5	15.2	13.9	12.5	11.2
100	15.7	14.4	13.0	11.6	15.4	14.0	12.7	11.3
100.5	15.9	14.5	13.1	11.7	15.5	14.1	12.8	11.4
101	16.0	14.6	13.2	11.8	15.6	14.3	12.9	11.5
101.5	16.2	14.7	13.3	11.9	15.8	14.4	13.0	11.6
102	16.3	14.9	13.4	12.0	15.9	14.5	13.1	11.7
102.5	16.4	15.0	13.6	12.1	16.0	14.6	13.2	11.8
103	16.6	15.1	13.7	12.2	16.2	14.7	13.3	11.9
103.5	16.7	15.3	13.8	12.3	16.3	14.9	13.4	12.0
104	16.9	15.4	13.9	12.4	16.5	15.0	13.5	12.1
104.5	17.0	15.5	14.0	12.6	16.6	15.1	13.7	12.2
105	17.1	15.6	14.2	12.7	16.7	15.3	13.8	12.3
105.5	17.3	15.8	14.3	12.8	16.9	15.4	13.9	12.4
106	17.4	15.9	14.4	12.9	17.0	15.5	14.0	12.5
106.5	17.6	16.1	14.5	13.0	17.2	15.7	14.1	12.6
107	17.7	16.2	14.7	13.1	17.3	15.8	14.3	12.7
107.5	17.9	16.3	14.8	13.2	17.5	15.9	14.4	12.8
108	18.0	16.5	14.9	13.4	17.6	16.1	14.5	13.0
108.5	18.2	16.6	15.0	13.5	17.8	16.2	14.6	13.1
109	18.3	16.8	15.2	13.6	17.9	16.4	14.8	13.2
109.5	18.5	16.9	15.3	13.7	18.1	16.5	14.9	13.3
110	18.7	17.1	15.4	13.8	18.2	16.6	15.0	13.4
110.5	18.8	17.2	15.6	14.0	18.4	16.8	15.2	13.6
111	19.0	17.4	15.7	14.1	18.6	16.9	15.3	13.7
111.5	19.1	17.5	15.9	14.2	18.7	17.1	15.5	13.8
112	19.3	17.7	16.0	14.4	18.9	17.2	15.6	14.0

Length/height (cm)	Boys' weight (kg)				Girls' weight (kg)			
	Median	−1 SD	−2 SD	−3 SD	Median	−1 SD	−2 SD	−3 SD
112.5	19.5	17.8	16.1	14.5	19.0	17.4	15.7	14.1
113	19.6	18.0	16.3	14.6	19.2	17.5	15.9	14.2
113.5	19.8	18.1	16.4	14.8	19.4	17.7	16.0	14.4
114	20.0	18.3	16.6	14.9	19.5	17.9	16.2	14.5
114.5	20.2	18.5	16.7	15.0	19.7	18.0	16.3	14.6
115	20.3	18.6	16.9	15.2	19.9	18.2	16.5	14.8

Table S4.2 Values for one standard deviation of NCHS/CDC/WHO reference median weight-for-height/length (49–115cm)

Length (cm)	One SD of median height (kg)		Length (cm)	One SD of median height (kg)	
	Male	Female		Male	Female
49	0.341	0.365	64	0.695	0.696
49.5	0.362	0.375	64.5	0.7	0.705
50	0.382	0.386	65	0.705	0.715
50.5	0.401	0.397	65.5	0.71	0.724
51	0.42	0.409	66	0.715	0.733
51.5	0.438	0.42	66.5	0.72	0.742
52	0.455	0.431	67	0.724	0.751
52.5	0.471	0.442	67.5	0.729	0.759
53	0.487	0.454	68	0.733	0.767
53.5	0.502	0.465	68.5	0.738	0.775
54	0.516	0.477	69	0.742	0.783
54.5	0.529	0.488	69.5	0.747	0.791
55	0.542	0.499	70	0.751	0.798
55.5	0.555	0.511	70.5	0.756	0.804
56	0.567	0.522	71	0.76	0.811
56.5	0.578	0.534	71.5	0.765	0.817
57	0.589	0.545	72	0.77	0.823
57.5	0.599	0.556	72.5	0.774	0.829
58	0.608	0.568	73	0.779	0.834
58.5	0.618	0.579	73.5	0.785	0.839
59	0.627	0.59	74	0.79	0.844
59.5	0.635	0.601	74.5	0.795	0.848
60	0.643	0.612	75	0.801	0.852
60.5	0.651	0.623	75.5	0.806	0.856
61	0.658	0.634	76	0.812	0.86
61.5	0.665	0.644	76.5	0.818	0.863
62	0.671	0.655	77	0.823	0.867
62.5	0.678	0.665	77.5	0.829	0.87
63	0.684	0.676	78	0.835	0.873
63.5	0.689	0.686	78.5	0.841	0.876

Length (cm)	One SD of median height (kg) Male	Female	Length (cm)	One SD of median height (kg) Male	Female
79	0.847	0.879	97.5	1.317	1.297
79.5	0.853	0.881	98	1.329	1.309
80	0.859	0.884	98.5	1.34	1.321
80.5	0.865	0.887	99	1.351	1.333
81	0.871	0.889	99.5	1.362	1.345
81.5	0.877	0.892	100	1.374	1.358
82	0.884	0.894	100.5	1.385	1.37
82.5	0.89	0.897	101	1.397	1.382
83	0.896	0.9	101.5	1.408	1.395
83.5	0.902	0.902	102	1.42	1.407
84	0.908	0.905	102.5	1.431	1.419
84.5	0.914	0.908	103	1.443	1.432
85	1.087	1.069	103.5	1.455	1.444
85.5	1.094	1.074	104	1.467	1.456
86	1.101	1.08	104.5	1.478	1.469
86.5	1.108	1.086	105	1.49	1.481
87	1.116	1.092	105.5	1.502	1.493
87.5	1.124	1.099	106	1.513	1.505
88	1.132	1.106	106.5	1.525	1.517
88.5	1.14	1.114	107	1.537	1.528
89	1.148	1.122	107.5	1.549	1.54
89.5	1.157	1.13	108	1.56	1.551
90	1.166	1.138	108.5	1.572	1.563
90.5	1.175	1.147	109	1.584	1.574
91	1.184	1.156	109.5	1.595	1.585
91.5	1.194	1.166	110	1.607	1.596
92	1.203	1.176	110.5	1.618	1.607
92.5	1.213	1.186	111	1.629	1.618
93	1.223	1.196	111.5	1.641	1.629
93.5	1.233	1.206	112	1.652	1.64
94	1.243	1.217	112.5	1.663	1.652
94.5	1.253	1.228	113	1.674	1.663
95	1.264	1.239	113.5	1.685	1.675
95.5	1.274	1.25	114	1.696	1.687
96	1.285	1.262	114.5	1.707	1.7
96.5	1.296	1.273	115	1.717	1.713
97	1.306	1.285			

Table S4.3 NCHS/CDC/WHO references expressed as percentages of the median by sex (49–115cm)

Length/height (cm)	Boys' weight (kg)				Girls' weight (kg)			
	Median	80%	70%	60%	Median	80%	70%	60%
49	3.1	2.5	2.2	1.9	3.3	2.6	2.3	2.0
49.5	3.2	2.6	2.2	1.9	3.4	2.7	2.4	2.0
50	3.3	2.6	2.3	2.0	3.4	2.7	2.4	2.0
50.5	3.4	2.7	2.4	2.0	3.5	2.8	2.5	2.1
51	3.5	2.8	2.5	2.1	3.5	2.8	2.5	2.1
51.5	3.6	2.9	2.5	2.2	3.6	2.9	2.5	2.2
52	3.7	3.0	2.6	2.2	3.7	3.0	2.6	2.2
52.5	3.8	3.0	2.7	2.3	3.8	3.0	2.7	2.3
53	3.9	3.1	2.7	2.3	3.9	3.1	2.7	2.3
53.5	4.0	3.2	2.8	2.4	4.0	3.2	2.8	2.4
54	4.1	3.3	2.9	2.5	4.1	3.3	2.9	2.5
54.5	4.2	3.4	2.9	2.5	4.2	3.4	2.9	2.5
55	4.3	3.4	3.0	2.6	4.3	3.4	3.0	2.6
55.5	4.5	3.6	3.2	2.7	4.4	3.5	3.1	2.6
56	4.6	3.7	3.2	2.8	4.5	3.6	3.2	2.7
56.5	4.7	3.8	3.3	2.8	4.6	3.7	3.2	2.8
57	4.8	3.8	3.4	2.9	4.8	3.8	3.4	2.9
57.5	5.0	4.0	3.5	3.0	4.9	3.9	3.4	2.9
58	5.1	4.1	3.6	3.1	5.0	4.0	3.5	3.0
58.5	5.2	4.2	3.6	3.1	5.1	4.1	3.6	3.1
59	5.4	4.3	3.8	3.2	5.3	4.2	3.7	3.2
59.5	5.5	4.4	3.9	3.3	5.4	4.3	3.8	3.2
60	5.7	4.6	4.0	3.4	5.5	4.4	3.9	3.3
60.5	5.8	4.6	4.1	3.5	5.7	4.6	4.0	3.4
61	5.9	4.7	4.1	3.5	5.8	4.6	4.1	3.5
61.5	6.1	4.9	4.3	3.7	6.0	4.8	4.2	3.6
62	6.2	5.0	4.3	3.7	6.1	4.9	4.3	3.7
62.5	6.4	5.1	4.5	3.8	6.2	5.0	4.3	3.7
63	6.5	5.2	4.6	3.9	6.4	5.1	4.5	3.8
63.5	6.7	5.4	4.7	4.0	6.5	5.2	4.6	3.9
64	6.8	5.4	4.8	4.1	6.7	5.4	4.7	4.0
64.5	7.0	5.6	4.9	4.2	6.8	5.4	4.8	4.1
65	7.1	5.7	5.0	4.3	7.0	5.6	4.9	4.2
65.5	7.3	5.8	5.1	4.4	7.1	5.7	5.0	4.3
66	7.4	5.9	5.2	4.4	7.3	5.8	5.1	4.4
66.5	7.6	6.1	5.3	4.6	7.4	5.9	5.2	4.4
67	7.7	6.2	5.4	4.6	7.5	6.0	5.3	4.5
67.5	7.8	6.2	5.5	4.7	7.7	6.2	5.4	4.6
68	8.0	6.4	5.6	4.8	7.8	6.2	5.5	4.7
68.5	8.1	6.5	5.7	4.9	8.0	6.4	5.6	4.8
69	8.3	6.6	5.8	5.0	8.1	6.5	5.7	4.9
69.5	8.4	6.7	5.9	5.0	8.2	6.6	5.7	4.9
70	8.5	6.8	6.0	5.1	8.4	6.7	5.9	5.0

Length/height (cm)	Boys' weight (kg)				Girls' weight (kg)			
	Median	80%	70%	60%	Median	80%	70%	60%
70.5	8.7	7.0	6.1	5.2	8.5	6.8	6.0	5.1
71	8.8	7.0	6.2	5.3	8.6	6.9	6.0	5.2
71.5	8.9	7.1	6.2	5.3	8.8	7.0	6.2	5.3
72	9.1	7.3	6.4	5.5	8.9	7.1	6.2	5.3
72.5	9.2	7.4	6.4	5.5	9.0	7.2	6.3	5.4
73	9.3	7.4	6.5	5.6	9.1	7.3	6.4	5.5
73.5	9.5	7.6	6.7	5.7	9.3	7.4	6.5	5.6
74	9.6	7.7	6.7	5.8	9.4	7.5	6.6	5.6
74.5	9.7	7.8	6.8	5.8	9.5	7.6	6.7	5.7
75	9.8	7.8	6.9	5.9	9.6	7.7	6.7	5.8
75.5	9.9	7.9	6.9	5.9	9.7	7.8	6.8	5.8
76	10.0	8.0	7.0	6.0	9.8	7.8	6.9	5.9
76.5	10.2	8.2	7.1	6.1	9.9	7.9	6.9	5.9
77	10.3	8.2	7.2	6.2	10.0	8.0	7.0	6.0
77.5	10.4	8.3	7.3	6.2	10.1	8.1	7.1	6.1
78	10.5	8.4	7.4	6.3	10.2	8.2	7.1	6.1
78.5	10.6	8.5	7.4	6.4	10.3	8.2	7.2	6.2
79	10.7	8.6	7.5	6.4	10.4	8.3	7.3	6.2
79.5	10.8	8.6	7.6	6.5	10.5	8.4	7.4	6.3
80	10.9	8.7	7.6	6.5	10.6	8.5	7.4	6.4
80.5	11.0	8.8	7.7	6.6	10.7	8.6	7.5	6.4
81	11.1	8.9	7.8	6.7	10.8	8.6	7.6	6.5
81.5	11.2	9.0	7.8	6.7	10.9	8.7	7.6	6.5
82	11.3	9.0	7.9	6.8	11.0	8.8	7.7	6.6
82.5	11.4	9.1	8.0	6.8	11.1	8.9	7.8	6.7
83	11.5	9.2	8.1	6.9	11.2	9.0	7.8	6.7
83.5	11.6	9.3	8.1	7.0	11.3	9.0	7.9	6.8
84	11.7	9.4	8.2	7.0	11.4	9.1	8.0	6.8
84.5	11.8	9.4	8.3	7.1	11.5	9.2	8.1	6.9
85	12.1	9.7	8.5	7.3	11.8	9.4	8.3	7.1
85.5	12.2	9.8	8.5	7.3	11.9	9.5	8.3	7.1
86	12.3	9.8	8.6	7.4	12.0	9.6	8.4	7.2
86.5	12.5	10.0	8.8	7.5	12.2	9.8	8.5	7.3
87	12.6	10.1	8.8	7.6	12.3	9.8	8.6	7.4
87.5	12.7	10.2	8.9	7.6	12.4	9.9	8.7	7.4
88	12.8	10.2	9.0	7.7	12.5	10.0	8.8	7.5
88.5	12.9	10.3	9.0	7.7	12.6	10.1	8.8	7.6
89	13.0	10.4	9.1	7.8	12.7	10.2	8.9	7.6
89.5	13.1	10.5	9.2	7.9	12.8	10.2	9.0	7.7
90	13.3	10.6	9.3	8.0	12.9	10.3	9.0	7.7
90.5	13.4	10.7	9.4	8.0	13.0	10.4	9.1	7.8
91	13.5	10.8	9.5	8.1	13.2	10.6	9.2	7.9
91.5	13.6	10.9	9.5	8.2	13.3	10.6	9.3	8.0
92	13.7	11.0	9.6	8.2	13.4	10.7	9.4	8.0
92.5	13.9	11.1	9.7	8.3	13.5	10.8	9.5	8.1
93	14.0	11.2	9.8	8.4	13.6	10.9	9.5	8.2

Length/ height (cm)	Boys' weight (kg)				Girls' weight (kg)			
	Median	80%	70%	60%	Median	80%	70%	60%
93.5	14.1	11.3	9.9	8.5	13.7	11.0	9.6	8.2
94	14.2	11.4	9.9	8.5	13.9	11.1	9.7	8.3
94.5	14.3	11.4	10.0	8.6	14.0	11.2	9.8	8.4
95	14.5	11.6	10.2	8.7	14.1	11.3	9.9	8.5
95.5	14.6	11.7	10.2	8.8	14.2	11.4	9.9	8.5
96	14.7	11.8	10.3	8.8	14.3	11.4	10.0	8.6
96.5	14.8	11.8	10.4	8.9	14.5	11.6	10.2	8.7
97	15.0	12.0	10.5	9.0	14.6	11.7	10.2	8.8
97.5	15.1	12.1	10.6	9.1	14.7	11.8	10.3	8.8
98	15.2	12.2	10.6	9.1	14.9	11.9	10.4	8.9
98.5	15.4	12.3	10.8	9.2	15.0	12.0	10.5	9.0
99	15.5	12.4	10.9	9.3	15.1	12.1	10.6	9.1
99.5	15.6	12.5	10.9	9.4	15.2	12.2	10.6	9.1
100	15.7	12.6	11.0	9.4	15.4	12.3	10.8	9.2
100.5	15.9	12.7	11.1	9.5	15.5	12.4	10.9	9.3
101	16.0	12.8	11.2	9.6	15.6	12.5	10.9	9.4
101.5	16.2	13.0	11.3	9.7	15.8	12.6	11.1	9.5
102	16.3	13.0	11.4	9.8	15.9	12.7	11.1	9.5
102.5	16.4	13.1	11.5	9.8	16.0	12.8	11.2	9.6
103	16.6	13.3	11.6	10.0	16.2	13.0	11.3	9.7
103.5	16.7	13.4	11.7	10.0	16.3	13.0	11.4	9.8
104	16.9	13.5	11.8	10.1	16.5	13.2	11.6	9.9
104.5	17.0	13.6	11.9	10.2	16.6	13.3	11.6	10.0
105	17.1	13.7	12.0	10.3	16.7	13.4	11.7	10.0
105.5	17.3	13.8	12.1	10.4	16.9	13.5	11.8	10.1
106	17.4	13.9	12.2	10.4	17.0	13.6	11.9	10.2
106.5	17.6	14.1	12.3	10.6	17.2	13.8	12.0	10.3
107	17.7	14.2	12.4	10.6	17.3	13.8	12.1	10.4
107.5	17.9	14.3	12.5	10.7	17.5	14.0	12.3	10.5
108	18.0	14.4	12.6	10.8	17.6	14.1	12.3	10.6
108.5	18.2	14.6	12.7	10.9	17.8	14.2	12.5	10.7
109	18.3	14.6	12.8	11.0	17.9	14.3	12.5	10.7
109.5	18.5	14.8	13.0	11.1	18.1	14.5	12.7	10.9
110	18.7	15.0	13.1	11.2	18.2	14.6	12.7	10.9
110.5	18.8	15.0	13.2	11.3	18.4	14.7	12.9	11.0
111	19.0	15.2	13.3	11.4	18.6	14.9	13.0	11.2
111.5	19.1	15.3	13.4	11.5	18.7	15.0	13.1	11.2
112	19.3	15.4	13.5	11.6	18.9	15.1	13.2	11.3
112.5	19.5	15.6	13.7	11.7	19.0	15.2	13.3	11.4
113	19.6	15.7	13.7	11.8	19.2	15.4	13.4	11.5
113.5	19.8	15.8	13.9	11.9	19.4	15.5	13.6	11.6
114	20.0	16.0	14.0	12.0	19.5	15.6	13.7	11.7
114.5	20.2	16.2	14.1	12.1	19.7	15.8	13.8	11.8
115	20.3	16.2	14.2	12.2	19.9	15.9	13.9	11.9

Table S4.4 NCHS/CDC/WHO weight-for-age references expressed as percentages of the median by sex (0–6 months)

Age (months)	boys weight (kg)				girls weight (kg)			
	median	<80%	<70%	<60%	median	<80%	<70%	<60%
0	3.3	2.6	2.3	2.0	3.2	2.6	2.2	1.9
1	4.3	3.4	3.0	2.6	4.0	3.2	2.8	2.4
2	5.2	4.2	3.6	3.1	4.7	3.8	3.3	2.8
3	6.0	4.8	4.2	3.6	5.4	4.3	3.8	3.2
4	6.7	5.4	4.7	4.0	6.0	4.8	4.2	3.6
5	7.3	5.8	5.1	4.4	6.7	5.4	4.7	4.0
6	7.8	6.2	5.5	4.7	7.2	5.8	5.0	4.3

Appendix S5
Statistics needed for anthropometric surveys

S5.1 Basic statistics

S5.1.1 Describing distributions

In any normal population there are variations in body shape and constitution between individuals. This can be illustrated by weighing all children that are one metre tall and plotting their weights on a graph. The graph will approach a bell-shaped curve, symmetrical around the median. This bell-shaped curve is called a Gauss curve or normal distribution curve. Although the shapes of the curve for each height are similar, the dispersion will be different. One curve will be more flat and wide, another will be more narrow and steep. This is the result of the variation of the weights of the children according the age groups to which they belong.

Figure S5.1 The distribution of weight for a population of boys who are all 91.5cm tall

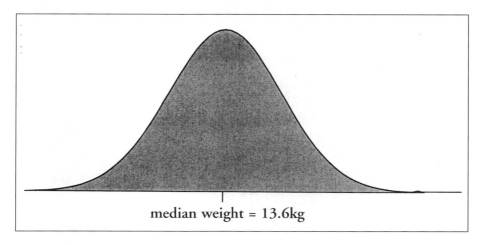

median weight = 13.6kg

This distribution can be summarised by presenting the mean or median (an average or central value) and the standard deviation (a measure of the spread of the distribution).

S5.1.2 The mean and median

A mean is calculated by summing all the observations and dividing by the total number of observations. So, the mean weight for the boys is calculated by adding all the weights and dividing by the total number of boys.

mean weight = <u>sum of all weights</u>
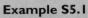
total number of boys

An alternative to the mean is the median. The median is the weight that divides the distribution in half.

Example S5.1
The weights for a sample of 11 boys is shown below:

ID number	1	2	3	4	5	6	7	8	9	10	11
Weight (kg)	13.6	12.3	14.7	12.8	13.2	15.1	14.4	13.9	13.0	15.2	12.6

The mean weight for this sample is calculated as

Mean = (13.6+ 12.3 + 14.7 + 12.8 + 13.2 + 15.1 + 14.4 + 13.9 + 13.0 + 15.2 + 12.6) / 11
     = 150.8 / 11
     = 13.7 kg

To obtain the median value, put the weights into ascending order. The weight that divides the sample into two equal parts is the median weight. This means there are the same number of observations above and below it.

ID number	2	11	4	9	5	1	8	7	3	6	10
Weight (kg)	12.3	12.6	12.8	13.0	13.2	13.6	13.9	14.4	14.7	15.1	15.2

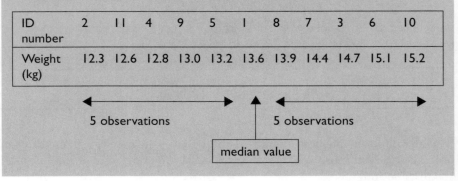

Note: For large sample sizes and distributions that are symmetrical (known as normally distributed) the mean and the median are equal. In nutrition surveys it is usually the median that is used as a central measure.

S5.1.3 The standard deviation

The spread of the distribution is described by the standard deviation. This is an average of the distance of each observed value from the mean, an average deviation. A simple average will not work because there are negative and positive differences and they cancel each other out, so the differences must be squared before they are added together. The square root is taken to get back to the original scale.

$$\text{standard deviation} = \sqrt{\frac{\sum (\text{observed value} - \text{mean value})^2}{(n-1)}}$$

where n = total number of observations (sample size)
and Σ = the sum of

Example S5.2
For the sample of 11 boys the mean was 13.7kg. From the observed values shown below the standard deviation can be calculated as:

ID number	1	2	3	4	5	6	7	8	9	10	11
Weight (kg)	13.6	12.3	14.7	12.8	13.2	15.1	14.4	13.9	13.0	15.2	12.6

$$\text{standard deviation} = \sqrt{\frac{\sum (13.6-13.7)^2 + (12.3-13.7)^2 + \ldots + (12.6-13.7)^2}{(11-1)}}$$

$$= \sqrt{\frac{10.47}{10}} = 1.02$$

The more variation in the weights in a population, the wider the distribution and the larger the standard deviation.

Figure S5.2 Distribution of weight for population of boys

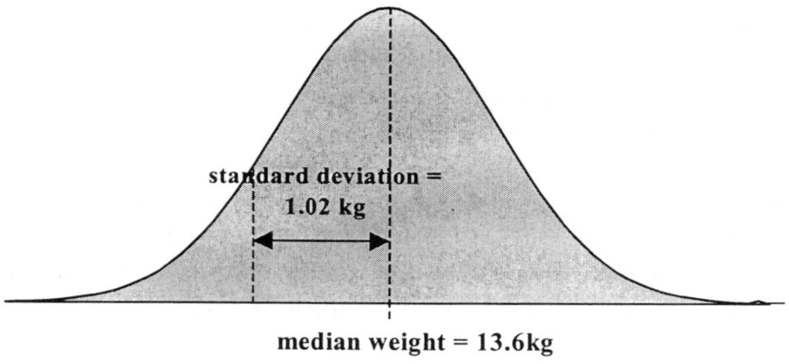

S5.1.4 Calculating a proportion or a prevalence

The prevalence, or proportion, of malnutrition is the number of children who are malnourished in relation to the total number of children in the sample. This is calculated by:

prevalence malnourished = 100 × number of malnourished children
                                            total number of children measured

> **Example S5.3**
> If a total of 908 children are measured and 101 children are found to be malnourished, the prevalence of malnutrition is
>
> prevalence malnutrition = 100 × 101
>   908
>
>   = 11.1%

S5.2 Confidence intervals and standard error

We study a sample to try to learn something about the population as a whole (without having to interview and measure the whole population). Usually we will want to estimate the characteristics of the whole population – eg, the proportion who are malnourished.

If we take a series of samples, the sample proportions would not be exactly equal to the true population proportion, but would be scattered around it. We need to know how large the error is between our estimate of the proportion and the real proportion. In other words, we need to know how precise (or accurate) our estimation of the true population value is.

Sampling errors (variability occurring because of chance) occur because we have observed only a section of the whole population. The larger the sample size that we take, the smaller will be the sampling error, that is, the more accurately (or precisely) we are likely to reproduce the characteristics of the population.

Another factor that influences the size of the sampling error is how variable the characteristic is within the population. If the variability of malnutrition is high, then we would expect the sampling error to be larger. If the variability of malnutrition is low, then we would expect the sampling error to be smaller.

The standard error of a proportion taken from a random sample is calculated as

$$SE = \sqrt{\frac{p \times (1-p)}{n}}$$

where p = proportion or prevalence
and n = sample size

If we took a series of samples from the population, the proportions that would be obtained would follow a normal distribution. Thus, the properties of normal distributions can be applied to the distribution of the sample proportions. For example, in one in twenty samples (five per cent) will the sample proportion depart from the population proportion (s) by more than 1.96 standard errors, that is outside the limits $p \pm 1.96 \times \sqrt{\frac{p \times (1-p)}{n}}$

Thus, the interval $d = p \pm 1.96 \times \sqrt{\frac{p \times (1-p)}{n}}$ will include 95% of repeated sample proportions.

However, in practice we only take one sample and only one sample proportion is obtained. Therefore there is a 95% chance (a probability of 0.95) of getting the sample proportion within the interval (d)

$$d = \pm 1.96 \, SE(p)$$

This interval is called the **95% confidence interval** (CI) of the estimate. It is a measure of the precision of the sample estimate proportion. The wider the CI, the less precise the results.

We say the probability that the CI contains the true population proportion is 95%.

Example S5.4
The prevalence of malnutrition was estimated at 9.5%.
The standard error is estimated at 1.17

$$
\begin{aligned}
\text{The 95\% CIs} \quad &= d = \pm\,1.96\ \text{SE(p)} \\
&= 9.5 \pm (1.96 \times 1.17) \\
&= 9.5 \pm 2.29 \\
&= 7.2\text{--}11.8\%
\end{aligned}
$$

S5.3 How to choose a random number

Sampling techniques rely heavily on the ability to choose a random individual, household or area to survey. Choosing a random number means there is no bias in selecting someone or somewhere to start a survey.

There are many ways to chose a number randomly; these include:

- drawing numbers from a hat
- using random number tables.

Both methods rely on giving an area/household/individual an identification number. Once the numbers have been randomly selected you can identify which area/household/individual has been selected by referring to your original identification list.

Drawing numbers from a hat or a bag

Determine the range from which you need a random number, for example 1–15. Then simply write down all the numbers on separate pieces of paper (you will have 15 pieces of paper in this example). Fold the pieces of paper and put them in a hat or plastic bag. Draw as many pieces of paper out of the bag or hat as you need. Each piece of paper that you draw out will have a number on it, representing a household or individual that you need to visit or measure.

Drawing numbers from a hat may be the simplest way to choose a random number. In addition, if you use this method, everyone will understand what you are doing. This method is obviously only practical if you need a relatively low random number – say below a hundred, as otherwise it will take you a long time to write down all the numbers on little pieces of paper and put them in a bag.

Using a random number table
Numbers can be read off with any required total numbers of digits. The steps involved in using this or any other set of random numbers are:

1. Decide on the direction in which numbers will be read – eg, left to right going down the page.
2. Specify the required numbers of digits. If a random number is required in the interval 0001 to 1342, four digits are needed (any of which may be zero).
3. Close your eyes and stick a pin (or other sharply pointed object) in the table (see page 286). Read off the required number of digits in the direction chosen in Step 1, starting with the first digit to the left of the point. If the resulting number falls within required interval, use this number. If not, repeat the process until an eligible number is drawn or move to the next number.

Random numbers

13118 50901 57493 96647 46146 65512 97571 49679 92251 36599
81111 33653 61544 90072 61635 94254 98222 49594 99403 56952
07124 56894 00475 09815 05299 17082 80775 11320 98562 68957
55155 23168 83063 80324 51450 68094 71844 68302 49552 12682
46406 44641 45461 75174 33268 86032 40355 58288 05532 29419
10616 17092 76614 04950 67982 28515 16782 86129 44391 64419
38497 57435 46124 37302 10783 93043 06903 77158 49638 26211
83203 45840 75843 75843 74567 75971 97779 98047 68916 35038
19236 62703 12863 14452 72228 55022 07024 43615 74802 02110
79024 60592 93692 29737 09314 26191 52484 11588 14078 85947
76073 57252 52795 67673 62267 29552 68244 49280 58583 42190
50568 66590 38807 30061 26336 46147 04554 44562 72604 63031
11838 73906 55981 23668 22627 88438 96686 73645 81410 10942
57618 30523 16757 11956 58411 41647 67884 30084 14500 66058
61846 47265 09508 11030 10462 93922 17022 7131 07827 94722
60935 25351 11687 07679 73455 58617 24415 56921 88450 50471
63328 21749 74262 77143 55995 50707 91516 38002 60552 00634
75937 07127 11014 00738 46159 09866 87587 41648 36538 24398
11981 89485 54965 08300 67724 24919 65682 50101 45470 07232
12311 17067 42758 64557 46297 28414 93801 81180 12176 08536
45160 76932 00433 42228 73696 27478 65321 22979 30198 86708
26427 48280 53441 44543 95231 39939 09251 09755 26671 89392
54568 17774 95705 28018 26507 63504 98872 22449 56423 59133
80855 94883 08969 16949 86045 68398 46164 57147 35104 37262
96203 73918 77875 48444 08167 58460 87945 52145 20330 77172
91210 89152 93904 27666 51080 00487 12073 41639 28717 33909
37808 11431 03351 82979 96677 41588 17592 5111x 84657 25427
47738 40686 00948 46598 99095 67011 05786 05642 26282 97486
03255 71561 78549 15611 49097 58375 70087 10066 83530 26684
92658 11755 39005 72386 20601 49630 85266 78939 89931 99674
86040 48908 88153 05616 91381 88378 28263 34725 80739 15251
87806 60615 14520 04557 72939 71060 10650 58769 07497 00808
46138 03111 47053 89391 83636 05877 17980 63940 23003 23737
81514 46994 77869 72054 22819 89316 77195 20194 65043 27706
28419 60216 07640 80670 84427 98368 99656 10214 04023 39899
99109 64711 06962 56790 96313 54470 18568 04319 31680 39507
15045 85129 03531 06107 93785 38290 00911 68388s 68686 53357
61398 94861 90462 09438 53920 59996 91957 39255 86563 20781
58455 18205 39389 18286 22994 78421 22241 04228 86679 47840
81025 70374 79493 39986 41707 57491 35647 43409 37182 73435

Appendix S6

S6.1 Example of an anthropometric data form with extra information

Survey district: _____ Village: _____ Cluster number: _____

Date: _____ Team number: _____

HH. no.	Child no.	Name	Age in months	Sex (F/M)	Oedema (Y/N)	Weight (kg) ± 100g	Height (cm) ± 0.1cm	WHM Registered in SFP/TFC (S/T)	Need to refer (Y/N)	Vaccination BCG Mark (Y/N)	Vaccination Measles yes with card = 1 yes but no card = 2 No = 0	Vaccination Vit A (Y/N/ DK)
	1											
	2											
	3											
	4											
	5											
	6											
	7											
	8											
	9											
	10											
	11											
	12											
	13											
	14											
	15											
	16											

S6.2 Example of a mortality questionnaire and data collection form using the current census method

Sample questionnaire

1. Who slept in this household last night?

2. How old is NAME?
    - ADD 1 to Total people in household
    - If under five add 1 to Total under 5 in household

3. Did anyone else sleep in this household last night?
    - If NO GO TO QUESTION 5

4. How old is NAME?
    - ADD 1 to Total people in household
    - If under five add 1 to Total under 5 in household

REPEAT QUESTIONS 3 and 4

5. How many children have been born since START DATE in this household?
    - ADD NUMBER TO No. of births since START DATE

6. Has anyone from this household died since START DATE?
    - If NONE then STOP
    - If YES ADD 1 to total deaths since START DATE

7. Was NAME under five years when s/he died?
    - If yes ADD 1 to No. < 5 deaths since START DATE

8. Has anyone else from this household died since START DATE?
    - If NONE then STOP
    - If YES, ADD 1 to Total deaths since START DATE

9. Was NAME under five years when s/he died?
    - If YES ADD 1 to No. < 5 deaths since START DATE

REPEAT FOR QUESTIONS 8 and 9

Sample data collection form for current census methods

Survey district: ——————— Village: ——————— Cluster number: ———————

Date: ——————————— Team number: ———————————

HH number	Total people in HH	Total under 5 in HH	No. of births since START DATE	Total deaths since START DATE	No. <5 deaths since START DATE
1					
2					
3					
.					
.					
.					

S6.3 Example of a mortality questionnaire and data collection form using the past census method

Sample questionnaire

1. Who lived in this household at START DATE?

2. How old was NAME at START DATE?
   - ADD 1 to Total people in household at START DATE
   - If under five ADD 1 to Total under-fives in household at start date

3. Is NAME still alive?
   - If NO ADD 1 to Total deaths since START DATE
   - If under five ADD 1 to Total under-five deaths since START DATE

4. Did anyone else live in this household at START DATE?
   - If NO GO TO QUESTION 7

5. How old was NAME at START DATE?
   - ADD 1 to Total people in household at START DATE
   - If under five ADD 1 to Total under five in household at START DATE

6. Is NAME still alive?
   - If NO, ADD 1 to Total deaths since START DATE
   - If under five ADD 1 to Total under-five deaths since START DATE

REPEAT QUESTIONS 4 to 6

7. How many children have been born since START DATE in this household?
   - ADD NUMBER to Total births since START DATE

Sample data collection form for past census method

Survey district: ——————— Village: —————— Cluster number: ———

Date: ————————— Team number: ———————————

HH no.	Total people in HH at START DATE	Total under 5 in HH at START DATE	Total deaths since START DATE	Total under-5 deaths since START DATE	Total births since START DATE
1					
2					
3					
.					
.					
.					

S6.4 Example of a mortality questionnaire and data collection form using the prior birth history method

Example of questionnaire

1. Have you ever given birth?
   - If NO, then STOP

2. When was your most recent birth?
   - If more than 5 years ago, then STOP

3. Was this before or after START DATE?
   - If after start of START DATE, then ADD 1 TO NEW BIRTHS since start date

4. Where is this child now?
   - If ALIVE, then ADD 1 TO CHILDREN AT RISK
   - If DEAD, then ask: did this child die before or after START DATE?
   - If child died after START DATE, then: ADD 1 TO NEW DEATHS, ADD 1 TO CHILDREN AT RISK

5. Did you have a birth before this child?
   - If NO, then STOP
   - If YES . . . repeat questions 1 to 5 for previous birth

Sample data collection form for previous birth history method

Survey district: _____ Village: _____ Cluster number: _____

Date: _____ Team number: _____

HH no.	Children at risk	New births since START DATE	New deaths since START DATE
1			
2			
3			
.			
.			
.			

Appendix S7
Statistics for the analysis of anthropometric and mortality results

The statistics needed to calculate the confidence intervals around either a prevalence of malnutrition or a mortality rate are similar. This annex shows how to make the calculations by hand and also by using two specially designed spreadsheets.

S7.1 Detailed calculations of standard error and confidence intervals for a prevalence

The standard error (SE) is relatively simple to calculate. There are two formulas: one for random sampling and one for cluster sampling.

S7.1.1 Random sampling

The formula for the calculation of the SE for random sampling is:

$$S.E. = \sqrt{\frac{p \times (1-p)}{N}}$$

Where, p = estimated proportion
N = sample size

Example S7.1
In a survey when 510 children were measured using random sampling, you estimated that the prevalence of acute malnutrition was 7.6%. The standard error would be

$$S.E. = \sqrt{\frac{0.076 \times (1 - 0.076)}{510}}$$

$$= \sqrt{\frac{0.076 \times 0.924}{510}}$$

$$= \quad 0.0117$$

$$= \quad 1.17\%$$

So, the 95% confidence interval, d, is equal to

$$
\begin{aligned}
d \; &= \quad \pm 1.96 * \text{S. E.} \\
&= \quad \pm (1.96*1.17) \\
&= \quad \pm 2.29
\end{aligned}
$$

Our 95% confidence intervals around the estimated prevalence of malnutrition are:

$$
\begin{aligned}
95\% \; \text{CI} \; &= \quad \text{estimated prevalence} \pm d \\
&= \quad 7.6 \pm 2.29 \\
&= \quad 5.3\% - 9.9\%
\end{aligned}
$$

Hence, in this example we would say that the prevalence of malnutrition was estimated at 7.6%, with 95% confidence intervals between 5.3 and 9.9%.

S7.1.2 Cluster surveys

The formula for the calculation of standard errors in a cluster survey is slightly more complicated:

$$\text{S.E.} = \sqrt{\frac{\sum (p_i - p)^2}{\{c * (c-1)\}}}$$

Where,
p = proportion of malnutrition in whole sample
p_i = proportion of malnourished in cluster i
c = total number of clusters

This looks complicated – but is easy to calculate if taken step by step.

Example S7.2
We will use real survey data from District A: 919 children were measured in 30 clusters.

To calculate $\text{sum}(p_i - p)^2$ make a table with six columns with your survey results in it:

Column 1   the number of each cluster
Column 2   the number of children in each cluster
Column 3   the number of children malnourished in each cluster
Column 4   the proportion of malnourished children in each cluster
Column 5   subtract the proportion of malnourished children in the total sample
(figure at the bottom of column 4) from the proportion of
malnourished children in each cluster
Column 6   square the figure in column 5 (multiply it by itself). Calculate the
total of this column.

Table S7.1 The calculation of the standard error for a cluster survey

1 Cluster c_i	2 Number x_i	3 Number malnourished y_i	4 Proportion malnourished P_i	5 Difference (p_i-p)	6 Difference squared $(p_i-p)^2$
1	32	5	15.6	−3.8	14.5
2	30	10	33.3	13.9	193.1
3	29	6	20.7	1.3	1.6
4	31	5	16.1	−3.3	11.0
5	31	4	12.9	−6.5	42.7
6	30	4	13.3	−6.1	37.3
7	30	5	16.7	−2.8	7.7
8	30	2	6.7	−12.8	163.1
9	30	9	30.0	10.6	111.5
10	34	8	23.5	4.1	16.7
11	30	2	6.7	−12.8	163.1
12	30	6	20.0	0.6	0.3
13	30	5	16.7	−2.8	7.7
14	34	3	8.8	−10.6	112.7
15	30	3	10.0	−9.4	89.1
16	30	7	23.3	3.9	15.2
17	30	4	13.3	−6.1	37.3
18	30	2	6.7	−12.8	163.1
19	30	7	23.3	3.9	15.2
20	32	4	12.5	−6.9	48.1
21	30	10	33.3	13.9	193.1
22	30	8	26.7	7.2	52.2
23	31	7	22.6	3.1	9.9
24	32	3	9.4	−10.1	101.3
25	33	3	9.1	−10.3	107.1
26	33	3	9.1	−10.3	107.1
27	34	10	29.4	10.0	99.5
28	31	9	29.0	9.6	92.0
29	30	14	46.7	27.2	741.4

1 Cluster c_i	2 Number x_i	3 Number malnourished y_i	4 Proportion malnourished P_i	5 Difference (p_i-p)	6 Difference squared $(p_i-p)^2$
30	29	12	41.4	21.9	481.4
all c	926 n	180 Y	19.4 P		3235.8 sum$(p-pi)^2$

In this example the standard error is:

$$\text{S.E.} = \sqrt{\frac{\sum (p_i - p)^2}{\{c \times (c-1)\}}}$$

$$= \sqrt{\frac{3235.8}{\{30 \times (30-1)\}}}$$

$$= \sqrt{3.719}$$

$$= 1.93$$

So, the 95% confidence interval (CI), d, is equal to

$$d = \pm 1.96 \times SE$$

$$= \pm (1.96 \times 1.93)$$

$$= \pm 3.78$$

Our 95% CIs around the estimated prevalence of malnutrition are:

$$95\% \text{ CI} = \text{estimated prevalence} \pm d$$

$$= 19.4 \pm 3.78$$

$$= 15.6 - 23.2\%$$

Hence, in this example from District A we would say that the prevalence of malnutrition was estimated at 19.4%, with 95% CIs between 15.6–23.2%.

S7.2 Using a spreadsheet to calculate the confidence intervals for a nutrition survey

The calculations for the standard error of a cluster survey are very time consuming. It is probably easier to do this in a computer program like Microsoft Excel. A spreadsheet has been designed for this and placed in the public domain. The spreadsheet is called 'anthropci' and can be found in the CD-ROM in this manual. Figure S8.1 shows you what the spreadsheet looks like – data from the example given above are shown (subsection S8.1.2).

Figure 7.1 Spreadsheet to calculate confidence intervals for a prevalence

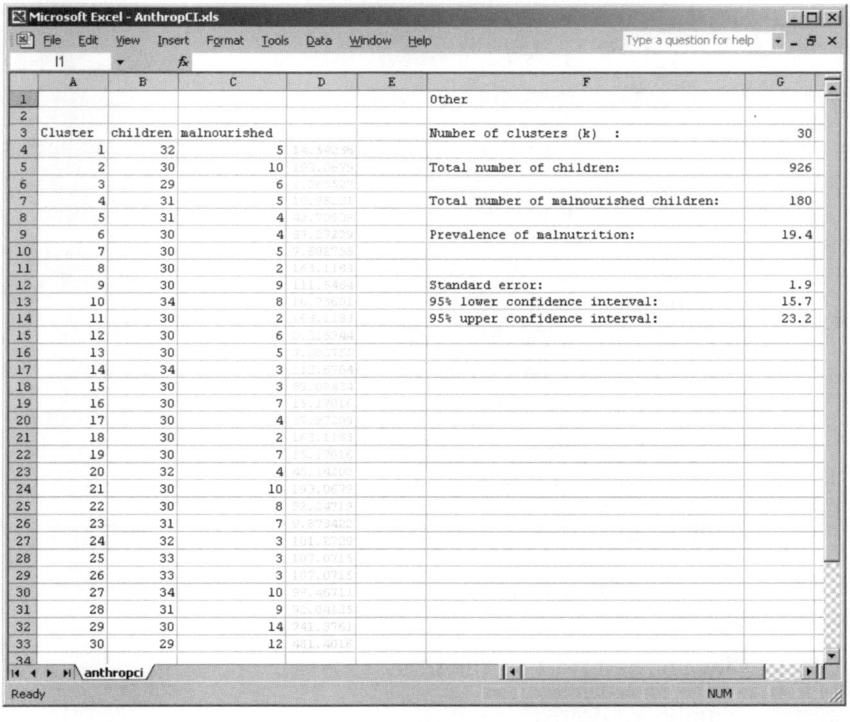

Using the spreadsheet is very easy:

- Enter the number of children per cluster in column B.
- Enter the number of malnourished children (don't forget to include the ones with oedema) in column C.
- The calculations are then made automatically for you and appear on the left of the screen in column G.

In this example, the prevalence of malnutrition was estimated at 19.4% with 95% CIs of 15.7–23.2%

S7.3 Calculating confidence intervals for a random or systematic mortality survey

The principles of calculating confidence intervals for mortality rates are exactly the same as those for the prevalence of malnutrition. However, you replace the *p* used in the formula with the proportion of deaths over person days at risk (PDAR) instead of the prevalence of malnutrition.

For example, the formula for the calculation of the SE for random sampling is:

$$SE = \sqrt{\frac{p \times (1-p)}{N}}$$

Where, p = estimated proportion
        N = sample size

Here p would be calculated differently for the past and current methods (see subsection C3.1.1):

For the current census method:

$$p \quad = \quad \frac{\text{Number of deaths during recall period}}{\substack{\text{Number of current residents} \\ + \frac{1}{2}\ (\text{number of deaths during recall}) \\ - \frac{1}{2}\ (\text{number of births during recall})}}$$

For the past census method:

$$p \quad = \quad \frac{\text{Number of deaths during recall period}}{\substack{\text{Number of residents at start of recall period} \\ - \frac{1}{2}\ (\text{number of deaths during recall}) \\ + \frac{1}{2}\ (\text{number of births during recall})}}$$

For the previous birth history method:

$$p \quad = \quad \frac{\text{Number of deaths during recall period}}{\substack{\text{Number of children at risk} \\ + \frac{1}{2}\ \text{number deaths during recall} \\ - \frac{1}{2}\ \text{number of births during recall}}}$$

S7.4 Using a spreadsheet to calculate the confidence intervals for a cluster mortality survey

The calculations for the standard error of a mortality cluster survey are time consuming. It is probably easier to do this in a computer program like Microsoft

Excel. Three spreadsheets have been designed for these calculations and they have been placed in the public domain. One spreadsheet has been designed for each of the three methods to estimate mortality in a cross-sectional retrospective survey:

- Current census method: *currentmethod.xls*
- Past census method: *pastmethod.xls*
- Previous birth history method: *pbh.xls*

The spreadsheets can all be found on the CD-ROM attached to this manual. Figures S7.2–S7.4 show you what the different spreadsheets look like. Note that the current and past census method programs have two spreadsheet pages each – one for CMR and one for U5MR.

Figure S7.2 Current census method spreadsheet (currentmethod.xls)

	A	B	C	D	E	G	H
1	Tallies					Other	
2							
3	Cluster	All people alive on day of survey	New BIRTHS	All DEATHS	#	Number of clusters (k) :	30
4	1	153	2	2	1.7E-08		
5	2	148	1	3	1.5E-07	Days since start event :	90
6	3	164	3	1	1.1E-08		
7	4	135	2	1	3.7E-09	Rate is per ... per day :	10000
8	5	158	1	0	9.7E-08		
9	6	161	2	4	2.9E-07	Rate Multiplier :	111.11
10	7	160	1	2	1.3E-08		
11	8	167	2	2	9.0E-09	New DEATHS recorded :	42
12	9	133	0	2	4.1E-08		
13	10	145	4	1	6.3E-09	New BIRTHS recorded :	68
14	11	152	3	1	8.0E-09		
15	12	149	2	3	1.4E-07	Mid-year population :	4579
16	13	159	3	0	9.7E-08		
17	14	147	4	0	9.7E-08	Proportion :	0.0092
18	15	201	3	2	6.5E-10	- Standard error :	0.0015
19	16	139	2	1	4.6E-09	- 95% LCI :	0.0062
20	17	153	2	0	9.7E-08	- 95% UCI :	0.0121
21	18	152	3	3	1.3E-07		
22	19	155	2	0	9.7E-08	Rate :	1.0191
23	20	150	3	2	1.9E-08	- 95% LCI :	0.6930
24	21	149	2	2	2.1E-08	- 95% UCI :	1.3453
25	22	153	1	0	9.7E-08		
26	23	140	2	0	9.7E-08		
27	24	177	3	3	7.0E-08		
28	25	144	2	0	9.7E-08		
29	26	157	0	2	1.5E-08		
30	27	155	1	0	9.7E-08		
31	28	154	3	4	3.3E-07		
32	29	145	5	1	6.5E-09		
33	30	137	4	0	9.7E-08		
34	OVERALL	4592	68	42	2.2E-06		

Microsoft Excel - MortalityCurrentHistory.xls
File Edit View Insert Format Tools Data Window Help   Type a question for help
USMR / CMR

Using the spreadsheet is very easy:

1. Enter the number of people alive at the time of the survey per cluster in column B.
2. Enter the number of new births in column C.
3. Enter the number of deaths in column D.

4. The calculations are then made automatically and appear in column H.

In this example the crude mortality rate (CMR) is 1.0/10,000/day with 95% CIs of 0.7–1.3/10,000/day.

Figure S7.3 Past census method spreadsheet (pastmethod.xls)

	A	B	C	D	E	F	G	H
1	Tallies						Other	
2								
3	Cluster	All people alive at beginning of recall	New BIRTHS	All DEATHS	#		Number of clusters (k) :	30
4	1	153	2	2	1.8E-08			
5	2	148	1	3	1.5E-07		Days since start event :	90
6	3	164	3	1	1.1E-08			
7	4	135	2	1	3.5E-09		Rate is per ... per day :	10000
8	5	158	1	0	9.6E-08			
9	6	161	2	4	2.9E-07		Rate Multiplier :	111.11
10	7	160	1	2	1.3E-06			
11	8	167	2	2	9.4E-09		New DEATHS recorded :	42
12	9	133	0	2	4.2E-08			
13	10	145	4	1	6.1E-09		New BIRTHS recorded :	68
14	11	152	3	1	7.7E-09			
15	12	149	2	3	1.4E-07		Mid-year population :	4605
16	13	159	3	0	9.6E-08			
17	14	147	4	0	9.6E-08		Proportion :	0.0091
18	15	201	3	2	7.4E-10		– Standard error :	0.0015
19	16	139	2	1	4.4E-09		– 95% LCI :	0.0062
20	17	153	2	0	9.6E-08		– 95% UCI :	0.0121
21	18	152	3	3	1.3E-07			
22	19	155	2	0	9.6E-08		Rate :	1.0134
23	20	150	3	2	2.0E-08		– 95% LCI :	0.6873
24	21	149	2	2	2.1E-08		– 95% UCI :	1.3395
25	22	153	1	0	9.6E-08			
26	23	140	2	0	9.6E-08			
27	24	177	3	3	7.0E-06			
28	25	144	2	0	9.6E-08			
29	26	157	0	2	1.6E-08			
30	27	155	1	0	9.6E-08			
31	28	154	3	4	3.3E-07			
32	29	145	5	1	6.2E-09			
33	30	137	4	0	9.6E-08			
34	OVERALL	4592	68	42	2.2E-06			
35								

Again, using the spreadsheet is very easy:

1. Enter the number of people alive at the start of the recall period per cluster in column B.
2. Enter the number of new births in column C.
3. Enter the number of deaths in column D.
4. The calculations are then made automatically and appear in column H.

In this example, the CMR is 1.0/10,000/day with 95% CIs of 0.7–1.3/10,000/day.

Note: In this example there is very little difference in the rates obtained by using either the past or the current birth history methods.

Figure S7.4 Previous birth history method: (pbh.xls)

	A	B	C	D	E	F	G	H
	Microsoft Excel - MortalityPBH.xls							
	File Edit View Insert Format Tools Data Window Help						Type a question for help	
	G36		fx					
1	Tallies						Other	
2								
3	Cluster	At risk	New BIRTHS	New DEATHS	#		Number of clusters (k) :	30
4	1	56	2	1	6.9E-09			
5	2	48	1	2	8.3E-07		Days since start event :	90
6	3	64	3	1	1.9E-11			
7	4	35	2	1	1.9E-07		Rate is per ... per day :	10000
8	5	58	1	0	2.7E-07			
9	6	61	2	2	3.5E-07		Rate Multiplier :	111.11
10	7	60	1	1	2.3E-09			
11	8	67	2	1	2.3E-10		New DEATHS recorded :	24
12	9	33	0	1	2.8E-07			
13	10	45	4	1	4.5E-08		New BIRTHS recorded :	68
14	11	52	3	1	1.5E-08			
15	12	49	2	1	2.8E-08		Mid-year population :	1573
16	13	59	3	0	2.7E-07			
17	14	47	4	0	2.7E-07		Proportion :	0.0153
18	15	57	3	1	4.5E-09		- Standard error :	0.0025
19	16	39	2	1	1.2E-07		- 95% LCI :	0.0104
20	17	53	2	0	2.7E-07		- 95% UCI :	0.0201
21	18	52	3	2	6.0E-07			
22	19	55	2	0	2.7E-07		**Rate** :	**1.6953**
23	20	50	3	1	2.2E-08		**- 95% LCI** :	**1.1564**
24	21	49	2	1	2.8E-08		**- 95% UCI** :	**2.2342**
25	22	53	1	0	2.7E-07			
26	23	40	2	0	2.7E-07			
27	24	77	3	2	1.3E-07			
28	25	44	2	0	2.7E-07			
29	26	57	0	1	6.9E-09			
30	27	55	1	0	2.7E-07			
31	28	54	3	2	5.3E-07			
32	29	45	5	0	2.7E-07			
33	30	37	4	0	2.7E-07			
34	OVERALL	1551	68	24	6.1E-06			
35								

`|◄ ◄ ► ►|\pbh /`   Ready   NUM

Again, using the spreadsheet is very easy:

1. Enter the number of children at risk per cluster in column B.
2. Enter the number of new births in column C.
3. Enter the number of new deaths in column D.
4. The calculations are then made automatically and appear in column H.

In this example the under-five mortality rate (U5MR) is 1.7/10,000/day with 95% CIs of 1.2–2.2/10,000/day.

S7.5 Population mean WHZ measurements

The mean WHZ is sometimes used to describe a population's nutritional status. This is calculated as:

$$\text{mean WHZ} \quad = \quad \frac{\text{sum of all WHZ}}{\text{number of children measured}}$$

Example S7.3
Using the survey data from District A, we can calculate the mean percentage WHZ of all the children in the sample. The sum of all the WHZ data was obtained by adding together the WHZ values for each child. So,

$$\text{Mean WFZ} \quad = \frac{-1233.77}{926} \quad = -1.33 \text{ z-scores}$$

You also need to present CIs for this value. You do this in much the same way as you calculate it for the prevalence (Section S7.1). Design a table like the one below:

Column 1   the number of each cluster
Column 2   the number of children in each cluster
Column 3   sum of WHZ for each cluster (add up each child's WHZ)
Column 4   mean WHZ for each cluster
Column 5   subtract the mean WHZ for the total sample (figure at the bottom of column 4) from the mean WHZ in each cluster
Column 6   square the figure in column 5 (multiply it by itself). Calculate the total of this column.

Table S7.2 The calculation of the standard error of mean WHZ for a cluster survey

1 Cluster c_i	2 Number	3 Sum WHZ	4 Mean WHZ m_i	5 Difference (m_i-m)	6 Difference squared $(m_i-m)^2$
1	32	−39.712	−1.241	0.091	0.008
2	30	−51.03	−1.701	−0.369	0.136
3	29	−35.873	−1.237	0.095	0.009
4	31	−44.857	−1.447	−0.115	0.013
5	31	−44.144	−1.424	−0.092	0.008
6	30	−40.02	−1.334	−0.002	0.000
7	30	−26.49	−0.883	0.449	0.202
8	30	−31.89	−1.063	0.269	0.073

1 Cluster c_i	2 Number	3 Sum WHZ	4 Mean WHZ m_i	5 Difference (m_i-m)	6 Difference squared $(m_i-m)^2$
9	30	−43.59	−1.453	−0.121	0.015
10	34	−44.812	−1.318	0.014	0.000
11	30	−30.99	−1.033	0.299	0.090
12	30	−43.02	−1.434	−0.102	0.010
13	30	−38.22	−1.274	0.058	0.003
14	34	−35.904	−1.056	0.276	0.076
15	30	−28.71	−0.957	0.375	0.141
16	30	−49.08	−1.636	−0.304	0.092
17	30	−43.62	−1.454	−0.122	0.015
18	30	−37.83	−1.261	0.071	0.005
19	30	−31.98	−1.066	0.266	0.071
20	32	−40.096	−1.253	0.079	0.006
21	30	−46.89	−1.563	−0.231	0.053
22	30	−46.02	−1.534	−0.202	0.041
23	31	−47.368	−1.528	−0.196	0.038
24	32	−42.496	−1.328	0.004	0.000
25	33	−33.726	−1.022	0.310	0.096
26	33	−38.511	−1.167	0.165	0.027
27	34	−54.706	−1.609	−0.277	0.077
28	31	−39.928	−1.288	0.044	0.002
29	30	−55.83	−1.861	−0.529	0.279
30	29	−46.429	−1.601	−0.269	0.072
30 c	926 n	−1233.77 total	−1.332 m		1.660 Sum$(m-m_i)^2$

Doing the calculations for the standard error of the mean is very time consuming. It is probably easier to do this in a computer program like Microsoft Excel, if possible, though there is no spreadsheet set up for this.

$$SE(p) = \sqrt{\frac{\sum (m_i - m)^2}{\{c \times (c-1)\}}}$$

$$= \sqrt{\frac{1.660}{\{30 \times (30 - 1)\}}}$$

$$= 0.044$$

So, the 95% CI, d, is equal to

$$d = \pm 1.96 \times SE(p)$$

$$= \pm (1.96 \times 0.044)$$

$$= \pm 0.86$$

Our 95% CIs around the estimated prevalence of malnutrition are:

$$95\% \ CI = \text{estimated mean WHZ} \pm d$$

$$= -1.33 \pm 0.86$$

$$= -2.19 \text{ to } -0.47$$

Therefore, in this example from District A, we would say that the mean WHZ was estimated at −1.33 z-scores, with 95% CIs between −2.19 z-scores to −0.47 z-scores. And you would fill in the results like this:

	6–59 months n = 926
Mean weight-for-height z-score	−1.33 z-scores (95% CI −2.19 to 0.47)

Appendix S8
Sample surveyor's manual and equipment list

S8.1 Example of a nutrition team member's manual for standard two-stage cluster anthropometric and mortality survey

The sample questionnaire forms which accompany this manual can be found in Sections S6.1 and S6.2.1 in Appendix S6.

General
This survey must be representative of the whole survey area, so every team must follow this method.

Arriving at the location (village or cluster)
Once you arrive in the location, try to find the location leader and explain why you are there. Once you have permission to undertake the survey, start as below:

1. Go to the centre of the selected locality (ask local people for information).
2. Randomly choose a direction by spinning a pencil or pen on the ground and noting the direction in which it points when it stops.
3. Walk in the direction indicated by the pen, from the centre to the outer perimeter of the locality, counting the number of households along this line.
4. Select the first household to be visited by drawing a random number between one and the number of households counted when walking. For example, if the number of households counted was twenty-seven, then select a random number between one and twenty-seven. If the number five was chosen, then the fifth household on the walking line is the first you should visit.

At the first house
1. At the house, introduce Save the Children and the purpose of the survey to an adult.
2. Start by doing the mortality questionnaire, then do the anthropometric questionnaire if necessary. Measure *all* children aged 6–59 months in the household.
3. The subsequent households are chosen by proximity. In a locality where there is a high population concentration, proceed by always choosing the next house to the right. Continue going to the left/right until the required

number of children has been measured and required number of households for the mortality survey. The same method should be used for all clusters. However, if the locality has a very spread-out population, then just proceed by choosing the nearest house. The nearest house is the one with the door nearest to the last house surveyed, whether it is on the right or left (this should save you a lot of time in an area where the dwellings are very spread out). Continue the process until the required number of children has been measured.

4. If there are no children under five in a household, do the mortality questionnaire, and then proceed to the next house.

5. All eligible children should be measured and weighed. This means that all children in the last house should be measured, even if this means exceeding the number required. If a child is not present at the time of the survey, go back to the house later to find the child (you should continue to look for the missing children until you leave the survey area). If you cannot find a child then you need to replace it with another, by continuing the sampling methodology. If a child has been admitted to an intensive feeding centre, the team must go to the centre and measure her/him there.

It is extremely important to follow this house-to-house method of selecting children if you are undertaking a random survey. If you simply call for children to be brought to the centre of the locality, it is likely that some of the children could be missed. This could result in bias. In addition to preventing bias, the house-to-house method also allows you to ask household questionnaires at someone's home, which makes it easier to verify what they are saying.

6. If you run out of houses to measure in a locality and have not found sufficient children (in this example, if you have not found 30 children) then you should proceed to the nearest locality. When you arrive at the nearest locality you should repeat the process of spinning a pen and randomly selecting a house to start at (Steps 1–4 described above). Proceed from house to house until you have measured sufficient children

7. If a child aged 6–59 months is not present when you visit a house, then make arrangements to visit the house later. You should make every effort to look for missing children until you leave the survey area.

> Randomness is the key to the success of the survey. Follow the above methodology as closely as possible. If a difficulty arises, then adapt the methodology as best you can, but remember randomness is the key. Record the change in methodology that you use.

Mortality questionnaires – based on the current census method

You need to get mortality information on the first 30 households you visit, whether or not they have any children aged 6–59 months. The procedure for the mortality questionnaires is described below.
1. Fill in all the general information (name of district, village, etc)
2. For each house ask the questions below to fill in the questionnaire form shown in Annex S6.2.1

1. Who slept in this household last night?

2. How old is NAME?
   - ADD 1 to Total people in household
   - If under five ADD 1 to Total under 5 in household

3. Did anyone else sleep in this household last night?
   - If NO GO TO QUESTION 5

4. How old is NAME?
   - ADD 1 to Total people in household
   - If under five ADD 1 to Total under 5 in household

REPEAT QUESTIONS 3 and 4

5. How many children have been born since START DATE in this household?
   - ADD NUMBER TO No. of births since START DATE

6. Has anyone from this household died since START DATE?
   - If NONE then STOP
   - If YES ADD 1 to total deaths since START DATE

7. Was NAME under five years when s/he died?
   - If yes ADD 1 to No. < 5 deaths since START DATE

8. Has anyone else from this household died since START DATE?
   - If NONE then STOP
   - If YES, ADD 1 to Total deaths since START DATE

9. Was NAME under five years when s/he died?
   - If YES ADD 1 to No. < 5 deaths since START DATE

REPEAT FOR QUESTIONS 8 and 9

Note: the questions for the other types of mortality questionnaire methods (the past census and previous birth history methods) can be found in Sections S6.3 and S6.4 in Appendix S6.

Children's anthropometric questionnaire
You need to measure at least 30 children. Fill in the children's form as you go from house to house. When you have measured 30 children there is no need to measure more though you should finish measuring all children aged 6–59 months in the household where the 30th child was measured.

Choosing the people to interview and measure
1. After you fill in the mortality data for a household, you should know if there are any children under five. So, ask for all the names of children aged 6–59 months. If a child's age is uncertain even after using the local calendar, then only children 65–110cm should be included. Any child outside these measurements should not be measured, unless their age is known for sure.
2. If a child is temporarily absent, ask the carer all the information about the child, arrange a return time and come back to measure the child. If a child in a selected household is admitted to a TFC, take details of the child (name, age, sex, which TFC, date of admission). You will need to measure this child in the TFC later.
3. Fill in the household number column. Remember that the household number should be the same for each house on the mortality and anthropometric questionnaires.
4. Then, for each child, fill in the data below:

Sex
Note the sex of the child by assigning an 'F' to females and an 'M' to males.

Oedema
Only bilateral oedema is considered to be of nutritional significance. Oedema can be diagnosed by placing a medium pressure (with a thumb) on the forepart of the leg (tibia) or on the upper side of the foot for three seconds. Oedema is present if a skin depression the shape of a thumb-print remains after the pressure is released.

The result is denoted by: N = absence of oedema, Y = presence of oedema.

Weight
The child is undressed and weighed on a Salter (25kg) scale. One of the assistants reports the measurement to the nearest 100g and the supervisor records this value immediately on the data collection sheet. The supervisor

repeats the value to the assistant in order to verify that the value was correctly recorded.

Height

Children aged above two years are measured in an upright standing position, whereas those younger than two years are measured in a reclined position. When age is difficult to determine, children measuring less that 85cm are measured in a reclined position and those measuring 85cm or above are measured in a standing position.

Measuring boards must be set on a flat surface and shoes must be removed. Feet must be placed correctly on the base of the board, with the child looking straight ahead.

As with weight measurement, the person conducting the measurements announces the value to the nearest 0.1cm and the supervisor records it and repeats the value for verification.

WHM

Calculate this index from the weight-for-height tables provided.

BCG

Check for the BCG scar on the child's upper arms. If the scar is present, record 'Y', otherwise record 'N'.

Measles

Ask to see the child's maternal and child health (MCH) card. Check the MCH card to see if a measles vaccination has been given. If the child has no card, or the measles vaccination has not been filled in the card ask the carer whether or not the child has had a measles vaccination. Try to make sure the mother understands you are talking about a measles vaccination, not polio, BCG or DPT3. Use the following code to specify the answer

1   = measles vaccination confirmed by card
2   = measles vaccination not confirmed by card, but confirmed by carer
0   = no measles vaccination.

Vitamin A status

Show the mother a sample vitamin A capsule. Ask the mother whether or not her child has received one of the capsules in the last six months.

Y   = yes, has received a capsule
N   = no, has not received a capsule
DK= don't know.

End of the day
Return to the houses where children were missed and try to find and measure them.

Check data-collection sheets completed by the teams. Has the data been correctly collected? Are there any values missing? Does any of the data appear to be erroneous? If so, go back to the household and double check.

S8.2 Example of equipment needed for a nutrition survey

	Item	Items per team	Total*
Weighing	Children's scales	2	12
	Hooks	1	6
	Poles	1	6
	Pairs of pants	2	12
	Standard weight	1	1
Measuring	Board	1	6
	Moving plate	1	6
Recording	Pencil	3	18
	Bic pen	3	18
	Eraser	3	18
	Pencil sharpener/razor	1	6
	Notepad (small)	3	18
	Clipboard	3	18
	Calculator	1	6
Other	Equipment bags for scales	1	6
	Document bag	1	6
Tents, etc	Blankets/sleeping bags	3	18
	Plastic sheeting	1	6
	Tents	1	6
	Cooking equipment	1	6
	Lamp	1	6
	Torch	1	6
	Insect repellent spray	1	6
	Water bottle	3	18

* this total assumes six teams

You will also need transport and fuel, money for per diems and letters of introduction from the local authorities addressed to the village leaders.

Appendix S9
Glossary of terms used in this manual

Acute malnutrition: reflects recent weight loss and is defined as **weight-for-height** <–2 z-scores or <80% weight-for-height median by NCHS standards and/or oedema, usually in children aged 6–59 months. This is also sometimes known as **global acute malnutrition**.

Agro-ecological zones: areas where the climate, physical environment and agricultural system are broadly similar.

Anthropometric measurements: body measurements such as weight, height and arm circumference which are used as a direct measure of an individual's nutrition and growth – their nutrition status. Collectively, the nutrition status of a population of children may be used for making comparisons over time or with other populations.

Anthropometric survey: a survey conducted to obtain a representative estimate of the prevalence of malnutrition.

Baseline data: a benchmark for analysis that depicts the nutrition status (and other resources, capacities and constraints) of a population in normal times, or before an intervention starts.

Bias: A consistent, repeated difference of the sample from the population, in the same direction; sample values that do not centre on the population values, but are always off in one direction.

Census: includes all the people in a population (in contrast to a survey).

Chronic food insecurity: a long-term inability of households to ensure sustained access to sufficient quantity and quality of food to live active and healthy lives.

Chronic malnutrition: reflects a height deficit and is defined as <–2 z-scores **height-for-age** by NCHS standards, usually in children aged 6–59 months.

Classification system: a system that establishes cut-off points using **percentages of the median**, or **z-scores**, and identifies different levels of nutritional risk.

Clean data: data that has been checked and corrected for mistakes or missing pieces of information.

Cluster sampling: the sampling technique that organises a **population** into smaller geographical areas for which the population size is estimated. Clusters are randomly selected from these geographical units according to their proportional population size. Individuals are then selected within each cluster.

Complementary foods: foods given to young children in addition to breastmilk or formula milk. Complementary food should usually be introduced into the child's diet at the age of about six months.

Confidence interval: an interval that has a specified probability of covering the true population value of a variable or condition.

Cross-sectional nutrition survey: a one-off assessment of the nutritional situation of a population, a 'snapshot in time'.

Current census method: a type of questionnaire used for conducting a retrospective mortality survey which begins by conducting a census of household members on the day of the survey.

Cut-off point: the point on a **nutrition index**, such as **weight-for-height**, used to categorise or screen individuals. For example, children below the cut-off point of 70% **weight-for-height** median are categorised as severely malnourished.

Distribution: a display that shows the number of observations (or measurements) and how often they occur.

Early warning: a process of monitoring indicators affecting livelihoods, with a view to warning of the threat of disaster ahead of time. This warning should normally trigger timely and appropriate preventive and/or mitigation measures.

Emergency: an extraordinary situation in which people are unable to meet their basic survival needs, or there are serious and immediate threats to human life and well-being.

Epi Info software: a series of microcomputer programmes produced by the CDC and WHO, for handling epidemiological data in questionnaire format, and for organising study designs and results into text and tables that may form part of written reports.

Exhaustive survey: a survey when the whole population is measured, or a **census**.

Food economy zone: a livelihood or food economy zone is a geographical area over which people pursue similar livelihood strategies such as agro-pastoralism. Food economy or livelihood zones are usually geographically distinct but may not be, eg, there may be a rice-farming zone covered with small zones where fishing is the main livelihood strategy.

Food security (insecurity): the ability (inability) of all people to assure themselves sustained access to sufficient quantity and quality of food to live active and healthy lives.

General ration: a basket of food commodities in a quantity sufficient to meet requirements (see **supplementary ration**).

Height-for-age: an index of past or chronic nutrition status; used to assess the prevalence of stunting.

Household: one person who lives alone or a group of persons, related or unrelated, who share food or make common provisions for food and possibly other essentials for living; the smallest and most common unit of production, consumption and organisation in societies.

Household economy approach (HEA): a qualitative approach to gathering information on household food security.

Hungry season or **hunger gap**: the period before harvests for agricultural populations, and before the rains for pastoral populations, when a population may not be able to access enough food.

Internally displaced person (IDP): persons or groups of persons who are forced or obliged to flee or leave their homes or places of habitual residence to avoid the effects of armed conflict, generalised violence, human rights violations, and/or natural or human-made disasters and who have not crossed an internationally recognised state border.

Live birth: Live-born children are defined as those born alive even if the child died immediately after birth. A baby who cried or breathed – if only for a few minutes – is counted as a live birth.

Local events calendar: a calendar that reflects important local events and seasons that might help a parent pinpoint the birth date of their child.

Malnutrition: adequate nutrition is the means by which people thrive, maintain growth, resist and recover from diseases, and perform their daily tasks. When nutrition is inadequate, people become malnourished.

Mean: the average value for a set of data, calculated by summing all the values, divided by the number of values.

Measurement error: the error that can result in a survey from incorrect (anthropometric) measurements being taken.

Median: a measure of central tendency, defined as the point above and below which 50% of the observations fall.

Mid-upper arm circumference (MUAC): a measurement taken on the mid-upper arm; used to assess total body muscle mass and, in some circumstances, acute malnutrition.

Moderate acute malnutrition: a child who has weight-for-height <-2 z-scores and $>=-3$ z-scores, or weight-for-height median <80 per cent and $>=70$ per cent, and/or oedema is moderately acutely malnourished.

Morbidity: a condition resulting from or pertaining to disease; illness.

Mortality rate: death rate; frequency of number of deaths in proportion to a population in a given period of time.

NCHS reference: growth percentiles developed by the National Center for Health Statistics in the USA, that provide standards for weight-for-age, height-for-age and weight-for-height.

Normal curve: a theoretical distribution of great significance in the statistics. Some of its major properties are (i) it is symmetrical and bell-shaped, (ii) the mode, median and mean coincide at the centre of the distribution, (iii) a fixed proportion of the observations lie between the mean and the fixed units of standard deviation.

Nutrition assessment: used in this manual to denote the entire assessment that is the anthropometric and mortality surveys and the qualitative assessment of the causes of malnutrition.

Nutrition index: when an individual's body measurements, such as weight, are related to age or height, and are compared with the measurements of a group of healthy people of the same height or age.

Nutrition indicator: a measure used at the population level to describe the proportion of a group below a cut-off point; example: 30% of the district's children are below −2 z-scores for height-for-age.

Oedema: the presence of excessive amounts of fluid in the intercellular tissue; the key clinical sign of kwashiorkor, a severe form of protein-energy malnutrition, carrying a very high mortality risk in young children.

Past census method: a type of questionnaire used for conducting a retrospective mortality survey which begins by conducting a census of household members at the beginning of the recall period.

Percentage of the median: a fraction or ratio based on a total of 100, where the median value of the dataset equals 100; a value that equals a proportion or part of a distribution where the median represents 100%.

Prevalence: the proportion of the population that has a condition of interest (eg, acute malnutrition) at a specific point in time; a value that is always between zero and one or expressed as a percentage.

Previous birth history method: a type of questionnaire used for conducting a retrospective mortality survey which involves asking mothers about children they have given birth to and whether they are still alive.

Protein-energy malnutrition (PEM): a range of clinical disorders occurring as a direct result of an inadequate diet and/or infectious diseases. The two extreme syndromes are marasmus and kwashiorkor. It should be noted that PEM is no longer a correct term to use, as nutrients other than protein and energy have a large part to play in determining the nutrition status of an individual.

Quantitative: quantitative methods are intended to measure the degree to which some feature of interest is present, such as the prevalence of malnutrition. Quantitative information can be collected using qualitative methods, eg, in an HEA assessment.

Qualitative: qualitative methods are usually exploratory and provide background descriptive information that may be used to describe relationships between points of interest, such as malnutrition and various causal factors.

Random sampling: the sampling technique that has a sample base available which lists every individual in the population and allows you to locate them. Individuals are randomly chosen from the list using a random number table.

Recall period: the period about which questions on birth and death are posed in a retrospective mortality survey.

Reference population: the group of healthy children whose measurements are used for comparison with those of individual children (see **NCHS reference**).

Representative sample: a subset of the population that is typical of the whole population.

Retrospective mortality survey: a cross-sectional survey in which questions are asked about birth and death during a period preceding the survey.

Sample: a part or subset of the population used to supply information about the whole population.

Sample size: the number of individuals or households to be included in the survey to represent the population of interest.

Sampling: the technique of selecting a representative part of the population for the purpose of determining characteristics of the whole population.

Sampling error: the difference between the results obtained from the survey sample and those that would have been obtained had the entire population been surveyed.

Sampling frame: the study population for which we need to know the estimate of malnutrition.

Screening: the practice of distinguishing between individuals who should be enrolled in a programme or intervention and those who should not be enrolled; a tool for identifying individuals at risk.

Secular trends: increases in anthropometric measurement between generations due to improved nutrition.

Severe acute malnutrition: a child who has weight-for-height <−3 z-scores or <70 per cent weight-for-height median and/or oedema is acutely malnourished.

Shock: used in this manual to refer to any event or process which contributes to the emergency situation.

Spring scale: a scale that measures weight by the amount a spring is pulled by the object being weighed; a hanging scale.

Standard deviation: a commonly used measure of variability, whose size indicates the dispersion of a distribution.

Stunting: reflects height deficit that develops over a long period of time and is defined as <−3z-scores usually in children aged 6–59 months.

Supplementary ration: foods that supplement the general ration to meet the needs of particular groups, such as malnourished individuals, young children, and/or pregnant or nursing mothers.

Survey: a method of gathering information about a large number of people by talking to, or measuring only, a sample of them; a way to collect information on people's needs, behaviour, attitudes, environment and opinions, as well as on personal characteristics such as age, nutrition status, income and occupation.

Systematic sampling: a modification of a simple random sample that consists of picking individuals or households at regular intervals from a random list or row of houses.

Underweight: a condition measured by weight-for-age; a condition that can also act as a composite measure of stunting and wasting.

Vulnerability: the degree to which an individual, household, community or geographic area is likely to be affected by a disaster. Vulnerability is also a risk of exposure to different types of shocks or disaster events, combined with the ability of the population to cope with these disasters or shocks.

Vulnerable groups: categories of people suffering from high degrees of risk. These may include, but are not limited to, women, children, elderly and disabled people, refugees, IDPs, food-insecure families and the poor.

Wasting: defined as weight-for-height <−2 z-scores or <80 per cent weight-for-height median by NCHS standards, usually in children aged 6–59 months; a condition that results from the loss of both body tissue and fat.

Weight-for-age: an index of weight in relation to age; it is not possible to determine whether a child who has a low weight-for-age is either stunted or wasted unless height-for-age and weight-for-height are measured.

Weight-for-height: an index of current nutrition status also referred to as wasting.

Z-score: a statistical measure of the distance, in units of standard deviations, of a value from the mean. The z-score is calculated by subtracting the mean from the data value and then dividing the results by the standard deviation.

Bibliography

ACC/SCN (1994) *Update on the nutrition situation*, Geneva.

ACC/SCN (2001) 'Assessment of adult undernutrition in emergencies'. Report of an SCN working group on emergencies special meeting in *SCN News*, 22, pp. 4–51, Geneva.

ACF (1999) *Nutritional status and food security evaluation in Korahi Zone, Somali Regional State.*

Action Against Hunger (2000) *Module 2: evaluating the nutritional situation*, a correspondence course.

Arimond, A. and Ruel M. T. (2003) Generating indicators of appropriate feeding of childen 6 through 23 months, *KPC 2000+*, Fanta, AED, Washington DC.

Bruce, J., Myatt, M. and Taylor, A. (2002) *Review of the sampling procedures analysis and interpretation of nutritional anthropometry surveys*, Unpublished report.

Buchanan-Smith, M. and Davies, S. (1995) *Famine Early Warning and Response – the Missing Link*, ITDG Publishing, London.

Cogill, B. (2003) *Anthropometric Indicators Measurement Guide*, Revised Edition, FANTA Project, USAID.

Collins, S., Duffield, A. and Myatt, M. (2000) *The assessment of adult nutritional status in emergency-affected populations*, ACC/SCN, Geneva.

Devereux, S. (2002) 'Poverty, livelihoods and famine', paper prepared for the Ending Famine in the 21st Century Conference, 27 February–1 March 2002, Institute of Development Studies, University of Sussex, UK.

Disaster Prevention and Preparedness Committee (1993) *National policy on disaster prevention and management*, Addis Ababa.

DPPC (2003) *Guidelines on emergency nutrition assessment*, Addis Ababa.

Fine, P. E. M., Donninghaus, J. M. and Maine, N. (1989) The distribution and implications of BCG scars in northern Malawi, *Bulletin of the World Health Organization*, 67(1), pp. 35–43.

Gibson, R. S. (1990) *Principles of nutritional assessment*, Oxford University Press, Oxford.

Golden, M. and Grellety, Y. (2002) *Population nutritional status during famine*, Paper presented at SMART meeting, Washington.

Kelly, M. (1992) 'Anthropometry as an indicator of access to food in population prone to famine', *Food Policy* pp. 443–454.

Kirkwood, B. R. (1988) *Essentials of Medical Statistics*, Blackwell Science, Oxford.

Lawrence, M. et al. (1994) 'Nutritional status and early warning of mortality in southern Ethiopia 1988-1991,' *European Journal of Clinical Nutrition*, vol 48, pp. 38–45.

Laws, S. (2003) *Research for Development*, Save the Children and Sage.

Maxwell, D., Watkins, B., Wheeler, R and Collins, G. (2003) Coping Strategies Index Field Methods Manual, WFP/Care.

MoH (1993) *Health and health related indicators*, Department of Planning and Programming in the MoH, Addis Ababa.

Moren, A, (1995) *Health and nutrition information systems among refugees and displaced persons*, Workshop report on refugees' nutrition November 1995, Nairobi.

MSF (1995) *Nutrition guidelines,* MSF, Paris.

MSF (1997) *Refugee Health: An approach to emergency situations,* Macmillan, London.

MSF (in press) *New nutrition guidelines*, MSF, Paris.

Myatt, M., Fekele, T. and Sadler, K. (2004), A field trial of a survey method for estimating the coverage of selective feeding programs, *Bulletin of World Health Organization* (forthcoming).

Myatt, M., Limburg, H., Minassian, D. and Katyola, D. (2003) 'Field trial of applicability of lot quality assurance sampling survey method for rapid assessment of prevalence of active trachoma', *Bulletin of the World Health Organization* 81 (12), Geneva.

Myatt, M., Taylor, A. and Courtland, R. (2002) 'A method for estimating mortality using previous birth history', *Field Exchange* Issue 17 Nov 2002.

National Center for Health Statistics (1977) 'NCHS growth curves for children birth–18 years', *United States Vital Health Statistics*, 165, pp. 11–74.

PAHO (1986) Tuberculosis Control, a Manual on Methods and Procedures for Integrated Programmes (PAHO Scientific Publication No. 498).

SACD-FAWR VAC (2003) *The Impact of HIV/AIDS on Food Security in Southern Africa.*

Save the Children UK (1999) *NSP results: Wolayita post harvest report – December/January 1999*, Addis Ababa.

Save the Children UK (2000a) *NSP results: Wolayita report – March/April 2000*, Addis Ababa, Ethiopia.

Save the Children UK (2000b) *The Household Food Economy Approach*, Save the Children UK, London.

Save the Children UK (2001) *Nutritional survey in Legambo woreda, February 2001*, Addis Ababa.

Save the Children UK (2004) *An analysis of Save the Children UK's Nutritional Surveillance Programme dataset in some of the most drought prone areas of Ethiopia, 1995–2001.*

Save the Children UK (2003), *Using Epi Info 6.04 Data processing and analysis of nutrition surveys. A training manual*, Save the Children UK.

Seaman, J., Clarke, P., Boudreau, T. and Holt, J. (2000) *The household economy approach: A resource manual for practitioners*, Save the Children UK, London.

Sen, A. (1997) *Poverty and famines: an essay on entitlement and deprivation*, Oxford University Press, Oxford.

Shoham, J., Watson, F. and Dolan, C. (2001) *The use of nutritional indicators in surveillance systems*, DFID technical support paper, ODI.

Toole, M. and Waldman, R. (1990) 'Prevention of excess mortality in refugee and displaced populations in developing countries', *JAMA* Volume 263 No 24.

Tomkins, A. and Watson, F. (1989) *Malnutrition and infection: a review*, ACC/SCN state of the art series nutrition policy discussion paper no 5, Geneva.

Tuan, T. et al (2002) 'Weighing Vietnamese children: How accurate are child weights adjusted for estimates of clothing weight?', *Food and Nutrition Bulletin* vol 23 no 4 (supplement).

The Sphere Project (2004) *Humanitarian Charter and Minimum Standards in Disaster Response*, Oxfam Publishing, Oxford.

UNHCR (2000) *Handbook for emergencies*, Geneva.

UN Standing Committee on Nutrition (2004) *Nutrition in Crisis Situations*, vol 1, Geneva.

Webb, P., Von Braun, J. and Yohannes, Y. (1992) *Famine in Ethiopia: policy implications of coping failure at national and household levels*, Research report 92, International Food Policy Research Institute, Washington DC.

WHO (1983) *Measuring change in nutritional status. Guidelines for assessing the nutritional impact of supplementary feeding programmes for vulnerable groups*, WHO, Geneva.

WHO (1985) *Energy and Protein Requirements. Report of a Joint FAO/WHO/UNU Meeting*, Technical Report Series 724, WHO, Geneva.

WHO (1995) *Physical Status: The use and interpretation of anthropometry*, WHO, Geneva.

WHO (1998) *Management of Severe Malnutrition: A manual for physicians and other senior health workers*, Geneva.

WHO (2000) *The management of nutrition in major emergencies*, WHO, Geneva.

WHO (2003) 'Nutrient requirements for people living with HIV/AIDS'. Report of a technical consultation'. Geneva.

Woodruff, B. (2002) *Review of survey methodology*, Presentation at SMART technical working session July 2002, Washington DC.

Woodruff, B. and Duffield, A. (2000) *The assessment of adolescent nutritional status in emergency-affected populations*, ACC/SCN, Geneva.

Young, H. (1992) *Food scarcity and famine: assessment and response*, Oxfam Practical Health Guide no.7, Oxfam, Oxford.

Young, H. (2004) *Nutritional Assessment: progress and remaining challenges*, Draft.

Young, H. and Jaspars, S. (1995) *Nutrition Matters: People, Food and Famine*, ITDG Publishing, London.

INDEX